TRANSFORM

TRANSFORM

Reclaim Your Body & Life From The Inside Out

MICHELLE ARMSTRONG

New York

TRANSFORM

Reclaim Your Body & Life From The Inside Out

Published in New York, New York, by Morgan James Publishing. Morgan James and The Entrepreneurial Publisher are trademarks of Morgan James, LLC.
www.MorganJamesPublishing.com

The Morgan James Speakers Group can bring authors to your live event. For more information or to book an event visit The Morgan James Speakers Group at
www.TheMorganJamesSpeakersGroup.com.

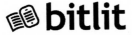

A **free** eBook edition is available
with the purchase of this print book.

CLEARLY PRINT YOUR NAME ABOVE IN UPPER CASE
Instructions to claim your free eBook edition:
1. Download the BitLit app for Android or iOS
2. Write your name in **UPPER CASE** on the line
3. Use the BitLit app to submit a photo
4. Download your eBook to any device

ISBN 978-1-63047-372-3 paperback
ISBN 978-1-63047-373-0 eBook
ISBN 978-1-63047-374-7 hardcover
Library of Congress Control Number:
2014945864

Cover Photo by:
Paul Buceta

Cover Design by:
Rachel Lopez
www.r2cdesign.com

Interior Design by:
Bonnie Bushman
bonnie@caboodlegraphics.com

In an effort to support local communities and raise awareness and funds, Morgan James Publishing donates a percentage of all book sales for the life of each book to Habitat for Humanity Peninsula and Greater Williamsburg.

Get involved today, visit
www.MorganJamesBuilds.com

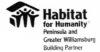

Habitat
for Humanity®
Peninsula and
Greater Williamsburg
Building Partner

This book is dedicated to my clients, past and present. Thank you for sharing your lives and opening your hearts with me. This book is a result of your awesomeness, courage, faith, and belief in yourself. You have inspired me on my own journey, and now you are an inspiration to all the eyes that read this book and the hearts it hopefully touches and opens.

CONTENTS

ACKNOWLEDGMENTS

Writing this book was not what I expected when the seed of the idea first entered my head. I thought this book would spill out of me in a few months. I did not expect it to take almost five years. Looking back, I can see now why it took as long as it did. I needed to undergo some transformation of my own in order to share this book in the way it is meant to be shared. This book was divinely guided, and the timing of this book is also divine. I have come to accept this reality: trust and allow the process to unfold as it is meant to.

I have many people to thank who have supported me with this book and who have encouraged me over the last five years. The first person is my dad: my number-one fan and my rock. Always supportive, continually encouraging, and never wavering in his love for me, words cannot express how much my father's presence in my life means to me. Thank you, Dad—for everything. I will love you to the end of time.

To my three editors (yes, there were three): to Aricia Lee, for once again streamlining my thoughts into poignant messages. To Amanda Rooker, whose editing abilities and loving and supportive approach to this book have made it what it is today. And to Suzanne Potts, who began this journey with me and whose patience, support, and intuitive guidance were so timely and paramount that I thank the grace of God for bringing Suzanne into my life. Thank you, Suzanne, for believing in me and being a partner and witness to the divine force behind this book.

I want to thank my clients who allowed pieces of their stories to be shared in this book, and who repeatedly busted my butt from week to week as to when I would finally finish this book. You are my inspiration, and I love you.

Thank you to Dr. Kristy Prouse for reviewing the appendix on hormonal health, and more importantly, her friendship and kinship. You are a beacon of light in this world! God bless you!

Thank you to Maureen "Mo" Hagan for so graciously taking time out of her busy life to peruse my manuscript and write the foreword. Mo, I will always be grateful to YogaFit® as the bridge that brought us together.

I am also enormously grateful to my wonderful little boy, who had to endure my absence on occasions when my head and focus needed to be elsewhere while I wrote this book, and during the moments of tears and my own personal challenges as I, too, transformed via this book. I love you to infinity and beyond buddy! Blast off!

I also want to thank photographer Dave Laus for the wonderful workout photos, Paul Buceta for the cover photo, nutritionist Kristina Graham for the twelve-week sample meal plan that appears in chapter 10, dietician Aimee Hayes for reviewing the nutrition sections, Matt Kahn for expanding my awareness, Donna McAuliffe-Edmonstone for being the best friend a person could ever have and for loving me unconditionally, my mum and brother for loving and supporting me, and my amazing and truly awesome agent Michael Ebeling for getting this book published and for paving a way of light and love for others. You are such a good soul, Michael Ebeling—thank you for being you! I also thank Morgan James Publishing for agreeing to publish this book and for repeatedly allowing me to extend my deadline not once, not twice, but many times. Thank you for trusting in the divine timing of this book.

Very importantly, I thank the divine love and gentle voice that speaks through and to me daily, who directs my footsteps and repeatedly lifts me up whenever I fall down (which has been often during the course of my life), and tells me often, "I love you, Michelle, and everything's okay," during times I have questioned and wondered. Thank you, God, for my extraordinary life! Thank you for all my shortcomings and strengths, and for all my challenges and hardships, which I now recognize as blessings and gifts through which I learn and grow. Thank you for using me to share with others your wish to see them achieve their potential and purpose in life, and receive the unwavering and unconditional love you have to offer them. I am grateful beyond words to be one of your teachers and messengers, and I pray this book becomes a gateway for others to experience and know what I have come to learn from you: that Love truly is the answer to everything, and that through divine Love and acceptance all things are possible for those who believe and are willing to receive, and who truly seek to transform into the extraordinary potential that's available to them.

Lastly, I also thank you, my reader, for choosing to read this book. Because of you, I get to be me. I can't express in words how much this means to me, but it means a lot.

In Love,
Michelle Armstrong

FOREWORD

by Maureen "Mo" Hagan

This is not a book about weight loss, nor is it an exercise program or diet regime. This book is about transformation. While it includes both nutritional guidelines for fueling your body and a workout program to guide you in your physical training, this book is fundamentally about how to create a radical change in how you think, what you believe, how you feel, and how you react—which, when understood and properly directed, inevitably causes major changes in one's life. In short, this book is a guide to help you develop a greater awareness of your mental, emotional, physical, and spiritual self, so that you can be transformed into the person you are destined to be.

My introduction to Michelle Armstrong occurred at a yoga training, and I was immediately captivated by her spirited and confident manner. As I have gotten to know Michelle, I appreciated firsthand her unique ability to communicate with people and, equally impressively, have them respond to her.

As an allied health and fitness professional with thirty-five years in the industry, I am very aware of how rare it is to find someone, like Michelle, who can train people and at the same time provide them with practical tools to put into action the ideas being taught. I also am the director of education for Canada's largest fitness education corporation and as such have hired and worked with thousands of speakers and educators during my twenty years with this company. After meeting Michelle, I jumped at the opportunity to present Michelle as a speaker at our conferences.

Michelle has been working in her chosen field of transformation for almost thirteen years and has personally counseled and trained hundreds of individuals. She has also spoken to thousands at conferences around the world, all with the goal of empowering those who are prepared to embark upon the journey of transforming their lives. Now Michelle presents, in this book, the techniques and tools she has developed over her career to allow the reader to identify and understand those self-sabotaging behaviors that prevent one from living the life he or she wants.

I am confident that whether you hear Michelle present, or you read and follow the guidelines in this book, you will realize, as have I, that unless you discover and start living your own personal truth, it will not matter if you are young or old, rich or poor, thin or obese, fit or out of shape; you will always be searching for something in your life outside yourself to bring you true happiness and peace. Michelle's experience and expertise will help you realize that what you are seeking is actually already within you, and all you need to do is transform the appropriate aspects of your inner world and behaviors to enable you to live the life you are really capable of having.

Every human being has the ability to change their current beliefs, emotional dependencies, thought processes, and physical abilities—or, in short, transform themselves. This book will show you, in a step-by-step manner, how to develop the proper mindset and to make the necessary changes.

Enjoy the transformation journey you are about to embark upon, embrace the results, and reap the many benefits of being the new you.

Maureen "Mo" Hagan, BScPT, BAPE
Award-Winning Fitness Instructor, Program Director, and Author

INTRODUCTION

At my weight-management and fitness studio, most clients come to see me because they are unhappy not only with their physical appearance, but with various other aspects of their lives as well, such as their careers or relationships. Their extra pounds—sometimes 100 pounds or more—are not just weighing on their body; they're weighing on their hearts and spirits. Many believe that if they can just lose the physical weight, they'll feel better about themselves, and life overall will be great. Perhaps you feel that way as well. If so, I can relate.

Five and a half years ago, I was fifty pounds overweight, and I had never felt so uncomfortable in my own skin. Today I am in my best shape I have ever been—I love my body, and I'm living my purpose and passion in life. But my journey here wasn't at all what I expected. I experienced what everyone else experiences—losing weight on the outside actually has a lot less to do with counting calories and exercising and more to do with healing what's not working right on the inside. I had to go deeply inward, even back to my childhood at times, to find the truth about why I was struggling with my weight at this time in my life, and dig deeply into my "heavy" stories, beliefs, thoughts, and emotions. Let me share with you a little about what I mean.

When I think back to my early childhood, only positive memories surface. I was born in Australia, but New Zealand was where I grew up. I call myself an Australian, but really I am a hybrid Australian and New Zealander. As a little girl, I experienced the world with a great level of love, awareness, and sensitivity. I was particularly sensitive to the energy of animals and nature, and I have felt a natural desire to bring love into situations of suffering for as long as I can remember. I was the sort of child who was forever bringing home stray animals, who would rescue and nurse back to life injured birds, and who just had to put a dying worm drying out in the sun onto a patch of grass to be restored and revitalized. I did not like to see needless suffering. I still don't. Sometimes my younger brother would tease me (as younger brothers do) by squashing ants with his feet, gleefully watching my horrified reaction.

According to my mum, I was a child who "sensed" things about people. I don't remember this in particular, but my mum told me I would often say some unusual things to her about guests in our home—people I'd never previously met. Overall, I had a deep sense of compassion as a child and I innately knew there was something magnificent and loving that coursed through me and held my sensitive world together.

In addition to my younger brother, I may as well have had three additional siblings, since I grew up spending a significant amount of time with my three cousins—the children of my mother's brother. We had barbecues and dinners together, went to the beach together, walked to and from school together, spent time together after school, and went on vacations that were always filled with fun, mischief, and adventure. The memories I have of these times evoke feelings of happiness, joy, and gratitude. I was cared for and loved, and my family was my world. It never occurred to me this might end. But it did.

I don't remember the exact moment I became aware of my parents' utter disdain and hatred for one another, but I do remember one minute feeling a part of a big, happy family, and the next minute watching it crumble down around me. My parents' divorce when I was twelve was, to put it mildly, a traumatic and chaotic affair. Not only did my immediate family disband, but my wider family disbanded also. I was left feeling confused, disillusioned, and alone. While I can look back now and see how unhappy my parents were and how emotionally ill-equipped they were at that time to cope with the demise of their marriage and their pain (never mind my brother's and my pain), I have compassion and understanding. But as a child I just saw my parents go from being two people I loved, knew, and trusted, to two people I thought were out of their minds and whom I no longer felt safe with or even recognized.

Somewhere amidst all the trauma and chaos, I lost myself in a cavern of despair and fear. By age fifteen I was out of the house, living in an apartment (I'd managed to get a lease by dressing up in a suit and lying to the landlord about my age). I was still going to school, and I worked several part-time jobs in the evenings. Some not so savory. I also had a pet cat named Monty who accompanied me everywhere I went, including on walks and in my car. Monty became my family, and I think Monty was as disillusioned as I was about life and his identity, since Monty thought he was a dog. By sixteen I was totally out of control and no longer cared one iota for my life. The pain of my family dissolving had turned from grief into anger and rage. I didn't know anymore where I fit in the world and the love and safety I'd felt in the world, I know longer felt or believed in and I took many dangerous risks at that time. It's a sheer wonder I'm still alive!

While I continued my relationship with God (which primarily took the form of begging and pleading with God to ease my pain and suffering), I simultaneously took little responsibility for my life and drowned my sorrows in alcohol. I sought comfort from food of the salty, sugary kind, and from love in all the wrong places. My body became a place of discomfort, and so I exited my body to avoid having to *feel*. I began to live only from the "neck up" and listen to and *believe* the stories my mind fed me, like "It doesn't pay to get too close to anyone because nobody can be trusted," "I'm not worthy of love," and "Life is safer being on your own since other people cannot be relied on." I came to believe the nonsense in my head as gospel, and the more I believed them to be true, the more problems showed up in my world as a result, and the more lost and bewildered I became. My world was crumbling, and I didn't give a shit because I felt totally alone and abandoned and life no longer had any meaning or purpose. I was full of anger and sadness, and I hated myself so much that I decided to embark on a downward journey of self-destruction. It seemed the only thing I knew how to do.

By the time I'd reached my early twenties (again, a miracle in itself), these destructive stories were all I knew. I was an emotional train wreck, angry at life and truly and completely out of control. Depression and anxiety had become my new best friends, and binge-drinking and binge-eating were weekly rituals and habits. My body had become a toxic warehouse, and the only time I ever acknowledged I even had a body was when it repulsed me from its reflection in the mirror. I'd verbally abuse it and then fill it with more alcohol and junk food to punish it. One time I remember looking at the back of my legs in a mirror and hating them so much, I threw what I think was a hairbrush at the mirror. "I hate you!" I screamed like a mad woman.

Ironically, even though my life was a total mess, I would still pray and dream of a better life—not that this would have been apparent from the outside, since I spent nearly every weekend getting smashed and then spent the weekdays eating my feelings of shame, self-loathing, and guilt. Sometimes I couldn't even get up the courage to go to work, I felt so bad inside. During these times I'd stay home and in bed, order some form of unhealthy takeout like pizza, and suffer in my own worthless misery. I could stay like this for days—in my room plagued with the constant chatter of absolute nonsense in my head, writing morbidly depressing stories in my journal, like: *My life is doomed. Life is full of darkness and deceit. I'm a target for abuse, and life is empty and meaningless; it has no purpose. Woe is me . . .* Yet there I'd also be, begging God to transform me because as unaware of myself as I was at that time, there was still a sense, somewhere deep inside my heart that there was more to life and more to me than what I was currently experiencing. I just didn't know how to achieve it. Maybe you can relate?

Then one day I woke up. Just like that, I woke from my nightmare. There was nothing dramatic or magnificent about it; I just woke up outside the chaos of my mind that allowed me to observe my mind, and see how what I was repeatedly thinking about and focusing on was impacting my life and I could change it, and I simply decided enough was enough. I was no longer going to continue to live my life this way. Who I was being was hurting not just myself but also other people. This was not the *real* me. What I felt as my truth, I was not living or exhibiting, and what love I knew I had inside, I was not receiving or giving. I was showing up instead as this angry, helpless victim in life, and I knew intuitively at that point that if I wanted my life to change and be better, the only person who could change it was me. I realized I had a choice. I knew in my heart I had a gift to give and a purpose to offer and share with this world. I knew that I needed to open up my heart again, surrender, and accept full responsibility for my life if I wanted to truly live as the person I knew I was *inside*.

The next several years of my life saw me participating in all sorts of different healing practices, modalities and therapies. I embarked full force on my quest to transform, and I opened the doorway again to *listen* to the divineness of life I'd once so naturally connected to as a child. I went to counseling and saw many different and wonderful therapists—all of whom helped me to go within and gain a deeper understanding of why I did the things I was doing and why I thought a certain way and believed the things I did. I went to numerous healing retreats and motivational seminars and workshops, and I became an avid reader of personal development books, absorbing every piece of learning I could find to help me understand myself better so I could free myself from the burdens that prevented me from being who I really wanted to be. I slowly began to release my limiting stories, and I embarked on a journey of truth, prayer, faith, surrender, love, and forgiveness.

In the process, I discovered the paradoxical nature of this journey toward healing. The more I took responsibility and humbled myself to dig around inside my mental and emotional body and let the darkness of my pain surface and release, the brighter the light in my world became. The more I started doing less and being still more, the deeper my relationship with God became, and the more my heart opened and love poured in and out. The more honest I became about the truth of what I was thinking and feeling in any given moment, the easier it became to manage my behaviors of binge-eating and drinking to excess. The more I understood the battle between my heart and my mind, the more compassion and acceptance I began feeling not just towards myself, but towards others as well. And the more transparent I became with myself and others, the less I experienced anxiety and depression and more peace and calm filled my spirit, allowing me to become more grounded and centered in my life. I could go on and on and on. The bottom line was that the more I looked inward rather than outward, the more quickly I transformed and the more fantastic my life became.

Since discovering how to transform myself from the inside out, my life's mission has been to help other people achieve the same. It's been a tremendous privilege to work with people at their most vulnerable and yet powerful times— those moments when they reach a crossroads and have to decide what kind of pathways and suffering they will choose to endure: the kind that results in continued misery for themselves and all the ones they love, or the kind that results from facing the truth of who they really are and changing from caterpillar to butterfly.

So although this book is about achieving the best body you can and the best health of your life, it's not a diet book or an exercise book—even though those topics are important and we will cover them in detail. This book is about transformation from the inside out. It's about awakening and becoming your greatest self! Experiencing true and lasting transformation will require you to go deeper than you have gone before or may even want to go. In fact, you already may want to run away screaming right now! But I can tell you from experience that going inward is the *only* path toward becoming the incredible being you were born to be and to achieve the body and health you want.

I consider it an enormous honor to be your guide on this journey. I've not only been through it myself, but I've also facilitated the transformation of over 600 men and women! And if I can do it, and if they can do it, my reader, so can you!

Here's a roadmap of the journey ahead:

Part One will guide you through a journey of self-discovery and profound awareness so you can uncover the hidden obstacles to losing the weight you want and living the life of your dreams! Here you will:

• Identify the "heavy stories" you live by that are manifesting your weight and health struggles.

- Learn to practice awareness to rise above the maze of your current struggles and connect to your inner wisdom so you can change what isn't working.
- Identify and reframe the beliefs, thoughts, and other "noise" that habitually weigh you down and trigger unhealthy behaviors.
- Learn how to truly love yourself and care for yourself accordingly.
- Address the obstacles of fear and unforgiveness.
- Create a practical action plan to bring the real, vibrant you to the surface!

One note about Part One. Because this inward journey can be littered with powerful roadblocks and resistance, I've structured each chapter in this part a little differently than the typical linear fashion. Think of a trail leading up a steep mountain that requires switchbacks, or reversals, in order to ascend. Sometimes it seems as if you're visiting the same point over and over again, or even backtracking. But if you took a direct path to the top, you'd never make it. It would be too steep and slippery, and you'd get injured or eventually give up. This slow ascent through switchbacks is actually the safest and most effective way to make it to the top. Similarly, we will intentionally circle through some topics in each chapter more than once in order to go one step deeper each time and help you get safely to your goal: the core of your true self.

Part Two addresses the physical part of your journey. After you emerge from the inner journey of Part One, connected to your inner wisdom and experiencing true self-love on the inside, taking care of yourself on the outside will become so much easier. But with all the contradictory diet and exercise advice out there, it's hard to know what eating healthy even means, and how to exercise to get the best results! So here you'll find the same guidelines I live by and teach to my clients: my Nutritional Guidelines and what I simply call The Workout. These are step-by-step, easy-to-follow nutrition and exercise guidelines and plans that are safe and effective for almost anyone. (Note: these recommendations are not intended to replace any specific advice from your doctor or health practitioner; as always, please check with them before beginning any new diet or exercise plan.)

At my studio, I consider it an enormous honor to work with women and men in the context of their mental, emotional, spiritual, physical health, fitness, and body issues, and to participate in their transformations. You will find pieces of their stories throughout the book. Because of the often intimate nature of the subject matters that arise within our transformation sessions, I have changed certain details to preserve my clients' privacy and the sacred relationship we share. In most instances, I have blended two or more client stories to highlight an insight or learning. However, in every case, the essence of their transformational journey has remained intact.

As the first step in our journey together, I'd like to show you how to do the centering meditation, which I practice regularly myself, teach my clients, and use as the basis of most of the practices and exercises in the book.

Centering Meditation

Step 1: Find yourself a space in your home that is quiet and where you will not be interrupted for five to ten minutes. You may even want to create a specific area in your house dedicated to your centering meditation practice so that your body and mind becomes accustomed to relaxing and centering whenever you are in this space.

Step 2: Sit in either a chair or on the floor. Sit in whatever way allows your spine to be as erect as possible and what provides you with the most comfort. Remove all sound and distraction and dim the lights if you can. Some people choose to light a candle; I like to use the battery-operated ones, as they give off a soft light and there's not potential of a fire hazard.

Step 3: Once seated comfortably (I recommend wearing comfortable clothes), close your eyes and pray and ask to be surrounded by Divine and Unconditional Love. During this step, you could place your hands on your heart, hold in them prayer position, or rest them gently in your lap—whatever feels right for you. There are no magical postures or words you need to use. Just maintain an erect spine as best you can, and ask to be surrounded by Love— and you will be.

Step 4: Keeping your eyes closed, begin to focus all your attention solely on your breath and the area between your two eyebrows. Imagine a white ball of light hovering gently in this area. Imagine this white light is the center of peace, and when you focus on the light you automatically become peaceful.

Breathe deeply in and out through your nose, expanding your diaphragm and belly as you inhale, and drawing your navel to your spine as you exhale. If your nose is blocked for whatever reason, inhale and exhale through your mouth. Do fifteen deep, long, and slow breaths, and on each exhale, intentionally and purposefully relax your body. Each inhale and exhale should be no shorter than five counts—more if you can manage.

Imagine that with each exhale, all tension, stress, and thought effortlessly leave your body. If you find you get an itch or thoughts start pouring into your awareness, simply keep breathing, focus more intently on your breath, scratch the itch, and observe the thoughts without giving them any direct attention, in the same way you might choose not to give your direct attention to the people's conversation in the booth next to you at a restaurant. Just like in the restaurant, you know people are talking around you, but you don't feel the need to tune into their conversations. You are more focused on what's happening at your table.

Step 5: After you've completed your fifteen deep breaths, allow your breathing to gently return to normal and draw your attention back to the white glow between your eyebrows. For the next five to ten minutes, keep your focus on the white glow, while simultaneously noticing your breath entering your body and leaving your body. With each inhale, feel more and more relaxed and more and more peaceful.

This completes the Centering Meditation. This practice can be done on its own as a longer, relaxing meditation, but for the purposes of this book, I invite you to begin each chapter with this Centering Meditation as described above. Now let's begin our inner journey with Chapter 1: Heavy Stories.

PART ONE

THE INNER JOURNEY

CHAPTER 1

HEAVY STORIES

When we awaken to the truth of our authentic self, the self that is limitless by nature, then we can decide what stories we want to keep and what new stories we want to be written.

When Rosemary walked into my wellness center, she had about eighty pounds of unhealthy body weight. Her motivation (a common one, I might add) was to see those three-digit numbers on her bathroom scale plummet as quickly as possible. As I do with all new clients, I began by asking Rosemary to tell me her "story," which revealed a wealth of valuable information as to why Rosemary was carrying the weight she had. Here is what Rosemary shared with me:

"I am a mother of three. I am married and I don't work. My husband has a really good job and we do very well financially. My husband doesn't notice I exist, and I pretty much do what he says to keep the peace. He often says mean things.

I try to ignore them. I am 44 and soon I will 45. I used to have some friends and now I have none. Social interactions are difficult for me. I feel old and I'm tired all the time. Taking my kids for a walk in the evenings is exhausting. They want me to play with them more but lately I don't feel much like playing. Nothing much interests me anymore. But I love my kids.

"As a family we normally go on vacation through my husband's work two, sometimes three times a year. We always fly, which I really don't like, as I'm claustrophobic and feel uncomfortable in the airplane seats. My body annoys and frustrates me. While I know I should be exercising more and probably eating differently, I don't have the motivation to do so. My husband also buys my clothes. I hate wearing them. I think I look awful. My husband and I don't have sex anymore. He's probably having an affair, but I don't care. I don't care much about anything anymore actually, except, as I said, my kids.

"I'm originally from London, England. We moved to California several years ago because of my husband's job. I have no family here, which isn't a big deal, since I'm not close with my family anyway. I miss England sometimes, but mainly I try not to think about it. I'm here because I think if I don't start doing something about my weight and my health I'll probably get sick, and then there'll be children who won't have a mother. My husband's a good father, I guess, but the kids aren't close to him at all. They are much more comfortable with me."

When I asked Rosemary about her childhood, she told me, "There's not much to tell, really. I was the youngest of eight. Nobody noticed I existed. Everyone was always busy doing things. I mainly just hung out by myself. Had a few friends—nobody special. And that's about it, I guess. I remain in contact with one of my sisters who now lives in Australia, but we're not close. I was an awkward child. I'm still awkward, I guess. I take anti-anxiety and anti-depressant medication, and sometimes I feel as I though I can't cope with my life anymore, and if nothing changes I won't be here next year. I'd like to come off the medication. I often feel lonely. And that's about it . . . my story."

I thanked Rosemary for sharing her story with me. And I then asked her if she could see any relationships between her story about herself and her challenges with her weight. I also asked if she could intuitively identify anything from her childhood that may have influenced what she is currently experiencing with her weight and health today. I like to ask my clients to share their intuitive thoughts. In many cases, clients doubt their own intuition, yet I have found them to almost always be correct.

I asked the question about Rosemary's childhood because our present experiences are always a reflection of our past experiences and the stories about ourselves that we have come to identify with. We bring all our stories, whether positive or negative, into every moment of our lives without being consciously aware of it. If we cannot tell ourselves a different story, then we will be forever locked inside one type of experience of life, and we are never free to show up in our lives any differently. We fail to recognize that there is more to us than the stories we repeatedly tell ourselves, and then we continue to repeat the story as though it's the only story we could ever experience. But just like a library, where you get to choose one book one week, read it, experience it, and then return it for another, you, too, can choose new stories in life if at any point you feel that the current story you are living and experiencing is losing its appeal and fulfillment. Not only is your story not *you*, but you are a writer of your story, not merely an actor following a script.

You cannot prevent the birds of sorrow from flying over your head, but you can prevent them from building nests in your hair.

Chinese Proverb

Over the next few weeks, Rosemary and I not only trained together physically, we also spent time talking at great length about all her heavy stories. We talked about all the beliefs and emotions she had wrapped up in each story, and how due to holding on to all these stories, Rosemary had *become* these stories, they were forming her identity, and they were making her fat and miserable.

We discovered that the primary heavy story driving many of Rosemary's stories was that she wasn't worthy enough to exist. As a result of her subjective interpretations and beliefs about her childhood—that her family never paid her any attention or affirmed who she was, which Rosemary eventually realized was about *them* and not about her—she realized that she has looked for her stories of low self-worth to show up in all her relationships, including her marriage. Rosemary realized that she contributed to "not being seen" by others through her own behaviors of withdrawing, not being social, not speaking her mind and truth, and not ever having an opinion or idea about anything. She became a wallflower to the world, even though inside she was screaming for attention—to be noticed, to be heard and to be loved. Over time this story manifested into more stories about her appearance. She decided she wasn't good enough for others because she wasn't attractive, was overweight, etc. Rosemary had lost her voice.

But the truth of the matter was that Rosemary was ignoring herself. It was Rosemary who chose to believe that Rosemary wasn't good enough and that she shouldn't exist. And as a result of her unhealthy choices, she had abandoned her body and was punishing herself by constantly feeding herself sugar and alcohol and never moving or exercising. Then when her body cried out in pain, in need of attention, Rosemary would shut it up quickly with medication. She realized her husband didn't go out of his way to ignore her, but rather she did everything she could to keep him at a distance. And why did she do all this? To prevent having to ever get close to anyone for the fear that they might hurt and reject her in the same way she felt her family had. And Rosemary didn't want to acknowledge this pain. So instead she chose at some level to become invisible. And the more weight she put on, the more she could hide the real Rosemary, on the *inside*.

When Rosemary entered the library of her mind and pulled out the stories she had about her childhood, they were depressing. When she rifled through the chapters she had about her twenties, *they* were all pretty miserable too. When Rosemary flipped through the pages of her engagement, her marriage, and her family situation to date, they were of the very same genre as the rest of her stories: misery, misery, and more misery. Then when Rosemary pulled out the big book about her identity, containing all the stories she had about who she was as a person, they were filled with chapters of sadness, depression, resentment, fear, and shame. Rosemary's encyclopedia of stories had such a "heaviness" about them that they were literally showing up in her body. There were few happy stories in

Rosemary's library, and even fewer possibilities for any future happy endings. If Rosemary was going to transform her health and body, she would need to find herself a *new* library, select some new stories and create new chapters in her life.

Thought Provokers

- *When you think back to your childhood, what stories immediately surface?*
- *Why do you think those stories/memories surfaced in your awareness right now?*
- *What feelings were evoked for you as you read Rosemary's story?*
- *Could you relate to some of Rosemary's stories?*
- *Can you relate to the feeling of not living your true self? If so, how does not living your truth make you feel?*
- *What is one story you know you have that is holding you back from being free to be who you want to be and live the life you want to live?*

We all have stories to tell. Your stories may be similar to or different from Rosemary's. But for each of us our stories serve to teach us something wonderful about ourselves we didn't previously know. It's only when we allow our stories to define us that they limit us, and we become trapped in the bodies and lives we don't want. But when we can rise above our stories, by recognizing that who we really are is the reader and *not* the content, and when we can heal the emotional wounds associated with our stories, only then will we set ourselves free. We will find it easy and effortless to take loving care of our bodies and to live the life we yearn for from our hearts.

Discovering Your Heavy Stories

If we let our automatic stories define us, we can be certain of an unfulfilling ending.

Before you can begin to write either a new chapter in your life or an entirely new book altogether, you first need to identify your current stories and how these stories are affecting and defining your current experiences. Our stories are the combination of our beliefs, thoughts, memories, ideas, and subjective opinions we create that form the lens through which we view ourselves and life in general, usually at a time in our lives when we are not fully aware that we are in fact the writers of the story and not merely the actors.

Even though many of our stories prevent us from living the life we want, we cling to our stories like life rafts. In truth, some of our stories can be more like backpacks filled with heavy bricks. These "heavy stories" tell us something negative about who we are as a person, and that are triggering and perpetuating our struggles with our weight.

As you discover and recognize your stories, you can then begin to make some specific correlations with your weight challenges and lifestyle, and then change the stories that no longer support the lifestyle and body you want to create. When you can see how your stories are limiting you from achieving certain results, you can *choose* to let go of these stories in the same way you would return a book to the library when you're done reading it. If you don't let go of the stories that define you, you will repeat your past into your future.

Here are some additional heavy stories my clients have shared with me over the years. Do you recognize any of these at work in your own life?

- My mother was an angry and selfish woman, and she never had any time for me. Therefore I'm not worthy or other people's time.
- My father was judgmental and critical, and nothing I did was ever good enough for him. I am not good enough.
- I've been fat my whole life, and that's never going to change. Why attempt to fix what can't be changed? I'll always be this way.
- Everyone treats me like shit. I'm the one everyone gets to dump on. It's not my fault. I can't help it.

- My ex cheated on me. People are liars. It's safer not to be in a relationship.
- I'm not smart enough to figure life out. I don't know what I want.
- I don't get any respect, and I'm not valued. I'm not important enough to be heard.
- I was forced to live in the limelight of my famous brother. I'm not worthy.
- No one is ever there for me. I'll never find love again. I am destined to be alone.
- I'm too old to start living my dreams now. I had my chance. It's gone.
- Everyone rejects me. Why bother getting close to people. I'm not good enough.
- I've always been used as the scapegoat. I have "sucker" tattooed on my forehead. If something bad is going to happen. It's going to happen to me.
- If I leave my current relationship nobody else will want me. Yes I've settled, but this abusive relationship is better than no relationship.
- Women use me. I'd rather have male friends than female friends. Women can't be trusted.
- I'm addicted to sugar, and I will never change. It's genetic.
- Nothing ever works out well for me. I always get screwed in the end so what's the use in trying anything different?
- I'm a loner. That's just how I am. Being alone is my destiny.
- If I don't take care of my mother, who will? There is nobody else but me!
- It doesn't matter if I try to lose weight, eventually I'll put it back on again. That's always been my pattern. Why would it change?

Your stories are a culmination of your beliefs, and they form the basis for why you engage in the behaviors that negatively impact your body, health and weight. The good news is that you are so much more than your stories.

Our Stories Are Our Teachers

Your unique stories are at the core of what makes you magnificent. If, for example, you were raised in a Christian home and your father was a pastor, then your stories will be different than those of someone raised in a Muslim home. If you experienced any type of major trauma in your life, then your stories will be different than those of someone who hasn't. If you were raised in Sydney, then again your stories will be different than those of someone raised in Jamaica. If during your childhood you were told to "eat everything on your plate or else," then your stories about *food* will be different from the child who was told to "eat only until you are full." If you were raised by a celebrity or a passionate athlete, then your stories about exercise and your body will be very different than someone who perhaps lost their legs during an accident and who was raised by their ailing grandmother. But what matters most is not the story itself, but rather what your stories can teach you about yourself.

If a story you're reading loses interest for you, why would you continue to read it?

We are each here on our own unique journey—and part of that journey involves uncovering and then living the *truth of who we are*. But who our true self really is often gets lost in the shuffle of our stories.

Sometimes our stories are pleasant and empowering—sometimes exciting, enlightening, even thrilling! But more often than not, for people struggling with their weight, their stories hold a lot of pain and suffering. Over time, they keep repeating their stories, and they eventually forget that their stories aren't telling the truth about *who* they are—limitless possibility, free to express our truth in any moment. In other words, they forget these are just stories, and they *become* the stories.

We can also develop an unhealthy relationship with our stories in the same way an abused woman might with her abusive husband. We tell ourselves that *we deserve our stories* and that any other story is a lie. Then finally we defend our stories, should anyone ever question them, because without them we won't know who we are.

When was the last time you were reading a novel and forgot you were the reader?

This "not knowing who we are" arouses intense feelings of fear and uncertainty, which nobody likes to feel. So instead we convince ourselves that our stories are real; the truth is *they are not real; they are just stories.* And when we forget that our stories are just stories, they form the boundary conditions of our lives and our experiences. They limit our capabilities and potential. They tell us: *I was overweight as a teenager, then again in my twenties—so now that I'm in my thirties, I'll be overweight just like I was before.*

Yet beneath all the stories you tell yourself about yourself is the truth of your divine and true nature. You are an extraordinary person, capable of being whoever you want to be in any moment. Someone who *knows* how to listen to your heart and who knows that you're not the "fit fat girl," as I once heard a client say, but someone living your purpose *as yourself* and treating your body with love.

Rosemary: The Sequel

Once Rosemary began to release her heavy stories, not only did she begin to lose weight, she literally transformed herself from the inside out. As she learned to trade out her heavy stories for more empowering ones, within ten months she went from being barely able to make eye contact or sit in a room with a stranger, to walking tall with her chest held high, making beautiful eye contact and confidently sharing truths about herself in small groups. Instead of being the wife who got ignored, she transformed into this sexy goddess her husband couldn't keep his hands off of. Instead of being too tired to walk with her kids, she became the mom who took her kids to Disneyland and who went for runs with them in the park. Instead of being the kid who was ignored during her own childhood, she became a woman who paid loving attention to the quiet person in the room. Instead of being the woman who used food to cope with her emotional pain, she became the woman who bought cookbooks and made healthy snacks at home. Instead of being the woman who was ugly and unattractive, she became the woman who was gorgeous and knew it! In less than a year, Rosemary became who Rosemary wanted to be—herself.

Our stories, heavy or not, can empower us when we view them as subjective interpretations of events in our lives that happened for a positive reason and purpose——*to teach us something wonderful about ourselves we didn't previously know*. Our past experiences happened for the purpose of *expanding*, not limiting, our lives. No matter what they are, how we may have interpreted them in the past, or what others have told us about them, the experiences that gave rise to our stories are never bad in and of themselves, because we have the power to interpret these experiences and tell our own stories about them that highlight the gift and opportunity to learn and grow spiritually. In this way, our stories serve to shape us and evolve us when we let them. Instead of backpacks of bricks, they can be hot-air balloons that take us to new heights beyond our wildest imaginings.

Practices: Heavy Stories

To begin your journey of transformation, you must begin with your stories. The following practices are designed to help you dig out all your stories and identify your heavy stories: the stories that are limiting you and fueling your challenges with your weight. You may use the journal pages at the back of this book, or you can use a separate journal of your choosing. As with all the practices I suggest in this book, they are best performed after the Centering Meditation provided in the introduction chapter, which will allow you to prepare for each practice and to go deeper.

Timeline

On the left-hand side of a page in your journal or the journal pages of this book, list every year since the year of your birth. Beside each year, as best you can remember, write down any significant and life-altering events. For example, you might begin with writing "my birth" next to your birth year, three years later you might write down that your sibling was born, two years later that your grandfather passed away, two years after that your house burnt down, and so on. You can write down every little event you can remember that held significance for you, and the more detail, the better. Note any injuries, major memories, divorces, weddings, accidents, movie screenings, vacations, mealtimes, school events, anything and everything that comes to your mind.

Then next to each of these events, write down what you've interpreted this event to mean about you and the world around you. For instance, if your mom constantly threatened to abandon your family and finally left in the middle of the night, as was the experience for one client of mine, then maybe your interpretation was also something similar to my client's: her mother's threats and eventual abandonment meant that "she was not lovable enough for her mom to stay." Finally, once you've written down how you interpreted the event and what you made it mean about you (not consciously of course), consider how it's now become one of your stories. Then ask yourself which of your stories are "heavy stories" that it's time for you to let go?

Letting Go

After you've completed the aforementioned exercise, open to a new page in your journal and simply write down your heavy stories as though you are being interviewed by a talk show host and they want to know, and you are willing to share, every intimate detail and memory of each of these experiences. Once your stories are written, read your stories individually as though you were somebody else. Then based on the awareness that you are not your stories, observe your stories as objectively as possible and write down any insights you have. Then as you review your stories, see if you can draw any correlation between your stories and what you are experiencing with your body and health, and in your life today. Also look for lessons and opportunities to be gained from your stories and how when you do, your life will be different in a positive way. Lastly, begin to write out some new stories, stories you would prefer to tell yourself and experience in your life.

CHAPTER 2

AWAKENING AWARENESS

Awareness is the ability to lovingly observe your mental and emotional activity without attachment or judgment, and to become present to that which wants to naturally arise within you to teach you something greater about yourself that you did not previously know.

W hen I met Lucy, she was carrying an excess of approximately fifty to sixty pounds on her body. Her presenting challenge was not her weight, but rather her inability to intentionally live fearlessly in her truth. Lucy knew deep inside herself that the way she was showing up in her life was not who she really was inside. On the outside, Lucy was an angry, fearful, distrusting, and resentful woman. Yet on the inside, Lucy was an intensely creative, loving, generous, kind, and deeply compassionate woman who genuinely wanted to make a difference in other people's lives. But Lucy didn't know how to live her truth—she was totally unaware of what was really going on inside her mind and what was fueling her current experiences and challenges with her weight. Lucy needed to develop a sense of *awareness*.

During our sessions together, Lucy was encouraged to inquire deeply into herself through the portal of her heart and really investigate at a deeper level the workings of her mind and her true feelings. After only a few sessions, Lucy was able to step outside herself and become an observer of her own mental and emotional activity and limitations. When Lucy became aware of herself—in that she was not only able to experience herself as herself, but was also more objectively aware of and present to herself as she was being herself—she realized that for her entire life she had never felt like she had "a voice." Because of the way she'd seen her mother silence herself and refrain from saying how she really felt to her father and her grandparents, Lucy learned to model her mother's behavior by keeping her own voice silent.

Lucy was experiencing what some call the "genetic curse," which is the automatic mental and emotional programming we inherit from our parents and then cement into our instincts by modeling ourselves in childhood after their behavior. This programming may have originated with our parents, they may have likewise received it from their parents, or it may be part of our genetic inheritance. But just because we have certain genetic predispositions or parental beliefs downloaded into our minds does not mean we cannot change our destiny—and changing our destiny begins with the simple act of *awareness*.

Awareness Begins with the Power of Now

Awareness begins with simply becoming *present to the moment you are experiencing*. It means not bringing into the current experience anything from your past. If the past creeps in, then the true experience of that moment is lost – and the ability to experience that new moment is gone. Living in the moment brings with it the truth of every moment that is peace, love, contentment, and joy. Just think of children under age five before they start to develop too much context and recall of past experiences. Each moment for them is a brand new and exciting experience. This is because they don't bring the past into the present. It's only as they get older and when the brain starts to develop that they begin storing memories and reliving those memories and the gift of the present loses its magic.

Being present to the now is also the key to becoming fully aware and discovering why you do what you do.

Through the eyes of the present moment, we can choose to rise up and view ourselves and our behaviors from a larger, grander perspective that reveals our power to make new and empowering choices. In fact, when I embarked on my own journey of transformation, this objective sense of awareness was my greatest discovery. When I was stuck inside the problems of my life, I was not able to see outside myself in a way that empowered me to make intentional choices and decisions. I was literally trapped inside the chaos of my mind, and it controlled me as opposed to me controlling it. Instead of being able to carve out the best pathways and directions for my life, my pathways were carved out for me. I wanted desperately to transform my experiences, but I simply could not affect any change at all because I was inside my problems, *being* my problems, instead of observing my problems as something outside myself from a grander, more divine perspective. Once I "awakened to awareness," my problems ceased to exist as problems, but rather presented themselves as opportunities. Awareness allowed me to release my own patterns of limiting behavior so I could fulfill my potential and be who I most wanted to be.

Imagine for a moment that you suddenly find yourself inside a large maze with walls so high you cannot see over them. You don't know how you got here, but you know you don't want to be in this maze, so you begin to run in fear, trying to find a way out. Because you cannot see what's around the next corner, you have to just run around aimlessly, hoping you'll stumble upon the correct path, the one that will help you get out of the maze so you can be free. Yet try as you might, you cannot find your way out, and so you continue aimlessly running around in circles, which is not only soul-destroying, but exhausting or you collapse in a heap and give up. All you want is to be free of the walls, free to know who you are outside of these walls, free to know what life really looks like beyond the walls of your self-imposed prison.

Now imagine another version of yourself who is able to float up out of the maze and take a bird's eye view. This you has the ability to see the maze in all its entirety. You can see how you entered the maze, what pathways will keep you trapped in the maze, and what route you need to take that will free you from the maze so you never have to feel stuck and trapped again.

Are you visualizing all this? Can you create an experience of this in your mind? *This* is awareness: the ability to be present in the moment, to rise above your experience, and to view yourself and your life from a new and grander perspective. Rather than leaving you feeling stuck, awareness helps you see new choices, which will ultimately allow you to navigate your life in the direction of what you want. This is why awareness is the first door we need to open if we want to have any control over our behaviors and actions. It gives us the perspective to see the entire puzzle of our lives, not just one or two of its pieces.

Awareness is the first door we need to open if we want to have any control over our behaviors and actions and ultimately our results.

Perspective Brings Peace

As you develop a sense of awareness—the ability to rise above the maze and take a grander view of your experiences—you can also experience the deep peace born of the love and wisdom that already resides in you. Awareness awakens that extraordinary, unconditionally loving, and wise part of your being that is able to observe you and your behaviors in a nonjudgmental and nonbiased way. This observant self has no preconceived ideas, expectations, or agenda about what you should and shouldn't be doing with your life. In fact, it has no preconceived ideas or agendas at all. It simply observes you and your existence from a place of love and contentment. It only wishes for you to come to know your greatest potential and realize your grandest experience of this life so you can then share this grandness with the world around you. Developing a relationship and communicating directly with this wise, loving, and aware part of ourselves allow us to enter into this state of awareness through the heart and discover the best course of action for us in any given moment—resulting in a deep peace that is beyond understanding and completely independent of your behavior or circumstances.

In this place of observant awareness, you are not emotionally attached to your stories or your beliefs anymore. Instead, you can observe everything that is happening within you without reactionary responses. In fact, you can observe your mind and behaviours with such attention and presence that you can literally and immediately change your mind and behaviors through your intention and heart-felt desire.

As you choose to dwell in this place of awareness, you will organically move into a higher and more empowering version of yourself that will allow you to outgrow and release old and limiting perceptions and experiences. Elevating yourself out of the maze of your mind and into a place of love, understanding, grace, and empowerment also brings with it a greater sense of appreciation and gratitude for all that you are. You will begin to see your problems and challenges as not really problems at all, but rather opportunities to be learned from, guided by, and appreciated. You will find yourself in the seat of creation where, through will and intention, you get to shape your own results and experiences of life.

Becoming Aware of the Divine

Awareness is not only a natural state of observation, wisdom, peace, and love, it is a powerful knowing that we are capable of achieving extraordinary things. We come to know in Awareness that we are never, ever alone. Awareness reminds us that we have an inseparable connection to the Divine from which we were formed, and that this connection has the power to heal any struggles we may be facing—including addictive behaviours, emotional pain, mental distortions and yes, weight gain.

As a connection to the Divine, awareness has the power to dissolve all problems and lift and release all emotional heartaches and suffering, while simultaneously revealing the gifts and learnings that will guide your soul to its greatest experience of itself. In this way, awareness brings comfort to suffering and love to fear. It allows you to release unwanted thought forms, express your emotions, and experience joy, no matter what is happening around you.

Awareness is the magic inside you that is going to relieve you from your emotional bondage to food and put a permanent end to your battle with your weight—if and only if you choose to embrace it and embrace a relationship with the Divine through awareness. Awareness allows you to see your greatest potential and reveal to you your true calling and purpose in life. Awareness has the power and intent to transform you mentally, emotionally, spiritually, and physically from the inside out.

Awareness is where fear cannot exist. It brings light to the darkness in our hearts and minds, and in our world. Awareness is love being aware of itself, and it is the key to your success, health and happiness. Awareness allows us to hear our intuitive and authentic voice and act on the nudges and whispers from God. It is the voice of your soul that aches to know and express itself through your deepest desires and heartfelt dreams.

THOUGHT PROVOKERS

- *Can you relate to the metaphor of the maze?*
- *Do you get trapped inside your head? How does this impact your life?*
- *Have you ever experienced a time and moment where you felt a deeper sense of being more aware and connectedness?*
- *What was this experience like for you?*
- *Are you aware of the feelings of others in relation to your behaviors and actions?*
- *What are some behaviors you know you have where you are unaware of why you engage in them?*
- *How different do you think your life would be if you could see over the walls and around the corners in your mind and thoughts?*
- *If you could see around the corners now, what behaviors would you choose to change and why?*

Experiencing Awareness

A question I am often asked is: "What does awareness feel like?" The only way I have found to explain awareness is to liken it to another experience. Have you ever had that kind of moment when, for just a brief second, time itself seems to stand still, and everything feels incredibly intense yet peaceful? Where everything around you is clear and vivid, as if all of a sudden, the mental activity in your mind silences and disappears and all that you can feel is a sense of awesomeness, truth, clarity, beauty, love, and peace?

You may have had this experience, as I did, when your beautiful baby was born and placed in your arms. You may have had this experience the first time you saw the man or woman you knew deep inside was the love of your life, or when you witnessed an awesome display of beauty, like a sunrise or sunset, animals in the wild, or the dancing of the Northern Lights. It may have occurred in a quiet moment when you suddenly became intimately aware of the wind rustling through the leaves of a tall, wise, old tree. Maybe you experienced an awareness of a greater reality when the soul of a loved one passed from this world to the next.

Often I can experience awareness when I close my eyes and turn my face up toward the sun. I simply become present to the warmth on my face, and that's all I need to still my mind—to come into the present moment and awaken to awareness. I am lifted out of my mental chaos and into the heart of inner quiet and bliss.

In these spectacular moments, when our breath seems to get caught in time and space, and our hearts seem to cease beating, we are experiencing what it feels like to be present and aware. It's like listening to the ocean and suddenly feeling that we are one with all that is. We know without needing to question how we know, that everything in life is happening exactly as it should and that we never have anything to fear. Awareness is to be at home with ourselves and a witness to ourselves as we journey through this experience called "life." Awareness reminds us of what is actually real—that love is all that exists.

Awareness Equals Freedom from
Unhealthy Weight and Health Issues

Weight issues inherently reflect a lack of awareness—we are simply unaware of what is really driving our unhealthy behaviors and actions. Hypnotherapists have posited that as adults, 95 percent of our motivations are unconscious. That means that we are only aware of why we do what we do 5 percent of the time! This is why even though we feel like we are in control of our lives, our thoughts and emotions, we find ourselves doing things we don't want to be doing. We are not what we believe, we are not our stories, nor are we what we think—we are not even our emotions. We are merely experiencing ourselves *through* these things. But only when we become aware are we able to make this powerful distinction between what we do and *who* it is we really are.

Developing awareness allows you to observe yourself and change in the moment the beliefs, behaviors, thoughts, and feelings that you know no longer serve you (which are usually rooted in our beliefs and heavy stories, as we discovered in chapter 1). Instead of getting off the sofa during every commercial break and searching inside the back of your fridge like it's the closet to Narnia, looking hopefully for that piece of sugary goodness that you know isn't there because you just looked ten minutes ago during the last commercial break, you will instead be able to lovingly and nonjudgmentally observe your insane behaviors (let's face it, it's true) and then intervene in this process of madness to carve out a new pathway for yourself.

Instead of feeling as though you're starving for a pizza, box of cookies, or salty, buttery popcorn, you will be aware of what is really driving your so-called pangs (i.e., your feelings) and be able to go deeper into the origins of these feelings to get to the truth of what is really going on within you. Once you shine the spotlight on the cause and not the symptom of your behaviors, you are dealing with the truth of the matter, and the truth, my friend, is what's going to set you free.

Your Life, Your Choice

The purpose of awakening awareness is simply to help you notice what is really happening in every moment so that you realize *you have the power to choose what happens in your life.* You can continue to live in the maze of your suffering, or you can choose to rise above it. —Your life is the way it is because of the choices you are making, regardless of whether they are fueled by pain and suffering. It is important that you know this and that you recognize right now that the only person who can change your life is you. Only you can stop yourself from picking up fast-food on the way home from work instead of making something healthy like a chicken breast with a quinoa salad at home. Only you can decide to go for a walk instead of going to the bar or watching hours of sitcoms. You have the power. In fact, you have more power than you realize—in fact, the purpose of this book is to help you realize that you can create the life and the body you want. You are strong and magnificent and I know you can do this. I believe in you and ask that you believe in yourself. You deserve to know the truth of who you are and hold hands with the power that surrounds you and is waiting to be awakened. Awareness is the key.

Practices: Awakening Awareness

One note before we continue: This chapter may have seemed a bit esoteric and less practical than the first chapter; this is because I have attempted to explain a state of being that is, well, in a way, beyond words. Similarly, the following practice may seem a little 'out there' at first glance. However, awakening awareness is a very practical and important step in your journey toward health and transformation, and you must learn to become aware of what's happening in the present moment at every level of yourself if you are to become aware of how to make new and empowering choices in every moment to make your life what you want it to be. Even if this practice doesn't make sense at first, I encourage you to do it *exactly* as it's written, as its benefit can only be known to you experientially. If you try to think your way through this exercise, or just read it rather than simply experience it, you will be unable to receive the deep benefits of this practice and the awareness and insight it brings.

Begin with the Centering Meditation from the Introduction chapter. Once fully and deeply relaxed, I want you to imagine there is another You capable of observing yourself from a nonjudgmental and loving place. Imagine that you are completely separate from yourself and you want to investigate this person called you. In particular, observe the following: any thoughts and beliefs (fixed ideas that we will discuss in more detail in the next chapter) that pass through your consciousness, any emotions that arise in your body, where they arise (e.g., the stomach), what color they would be if they were a color, and what messages they hold for you in their wisdom. Observe any physical sensations in your body. Do you feel tightness or tension, nausea, or twitching? Where do you feel these sensations, and again, what messages do they hold for you in their wisdom? After a few minutes of doing this, become *aware* of that which is *aware* of you being *aware*. Yes, I know how this sounds. But you're going to have to trust me. If at first you aren't able to become aware of that which is aware of you being aware, don't just give up and say, "oh well, that didn't work" but instead *keep practicing*. You will get it eventually, and when you do, so many light bulbs will go off in your head that you'll wonder how it was you could not possibly have been aware of this experience before.

CHAPTER 3

BELIEVING IS SEEING

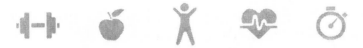

You can expect to experience in your life what you believe.

When Trudy walked through my studio doors, she was full of optimism about transforming her body. She was fast approaching her fortieth birthday and had decided this was going to be her turning point. She had put on an extra fifty pounds of fat when she was pregnant in her late twenties, and had assumed the pounds would simply fall away after she had the kids, but they never did. Now she had decided that enough was enough. She needed to do something.

Trudy's enthusiasm was impressive . . . at first. She had agreed to train with me three times a week and alter her diet to cut out all alcohol, unhealthy fats, processed foods, and sugar. She shared with me that this was going to be a challenge, but when she set her mind to do something, she got things done!

Trudy was committed, determined, passionate, and gung ho. I could almost see a cape with the words "Super Woman" flying out from behind her.

But after two weeks of training as planned, Trudy had not lost more than two pounds. She should easily have lost between four and six pounds with the regimen she was on, so this immediately raised a red flag. As much as Trudy was singing a good tune, her results weren't reflecting her intention. I could see the familiar face of discouragement starting to settle in on her and the all-too-common appearance of defeat. So we did what I do with all my clients when their progress doesn't reflect what it should. I sat Trudy down, looked her square in the eyeballs, and said, "Girl, we need to talk."

What we *want* and what we *believe* can often be two very different things.

As I began my typical inquiry into Trudy's mental and emotional world, I began to bring to the surface some deeply entrenched beliefs that were not in alignment with Trudy's attempts to transform. They were as follows:

- Trudy had been overweight her whole life and had tried several times before to lose weight with no long-term success. She confessed that while she wanted something different, she couldn't help but believe that this time would probably be no different.
- She said she enjoyed our workouts, but she "didn't have the time" to exercise outside our sessions.
- She said she "needed" sugar to survive and help her get through her day. If she had to stop eating sugar, then she wouldn't perform well at work and that would be a disaster.
- She confessed she was still drinking one to two glasses of red wine a day because "surely one to two glasses a night wouldn't make that much difference" to her weight. Plus red wine is actually good for you—good for the heart, apparently—so *No*, she was not willing to give up the booze.
- She said it was not possible to eat healthy at nighttime because her husband liked eating junk food, and since he was the one who brought all the junk food into the house, she couldn't avoid it and stop from eating it.

- She said sweets and snacks helped her calm down, and she "didn't have the time" to meditate and "go within."

When I heard these beliefs, it was no surprise to me at all why Trudy was not seeing the results she'd hoped for. She had too many limiting beliefs that ran counter to her desires and intentions. But when we began to unravel and then reframe her beliefs and perceptions, Trudy began to see how what she *believed* directly impacted the results she was experiencing. Even better, when she took on some new and empowering beliefs that were aligned with her intentions and goals, she began to see the results she wanted. She was shocked at the power her beliefs had over her behaviors.

A belief is not merely an idea the mind possesses; it is an idea that possesses the mind.
Robert Oxton Bolt

What Is a Belief?

A belief is a thought or idea that's been confirmed over time through our life experiences. Ironically, our beliefs become self-fulfilling prophecies because of the way our brains work. Regardless of whether the belief is true or not, the brain will seek to prove our belief is true on the inside by filtering out any experience that does not match our belief, and that match out beliefs on the outside. The problem is that although we get in life what we look for, this may not always be what we want.

Most of our deepest beliefs were adopted *unconsciously*, meaning we didn't even have full awareness that we were forming our beliefs and life views at the time they were being downloaded into our nervous system. Much like a computer downloads software, we download the majority of our beliefs during childhood from those around us, including parents, older siblings, grandparents, teachers, religious leaders, and the media—beliefs that they, too, unconsciously downloaded at some point from their own childhood influences, unique experiences, and views of the world.

Believing Has Its Pros and Cons

It's important to recognize that 1) beliefs are entirely subjective, and 2) your beliefs determine your experience. Therefore, what you *believe* is what you will experience in your life, which was the undesirable result for Trudy. But the good news is you can also choose what you want to believe the moment you become *aware* (see chapter 2) and realize that you have the power to choose. You don't have to live by the beliefs of another person or persons. Or the beliefs held by society. Nor do you have to continue to believe the ideas in your head that run counter to the results you wish to experience. Instead, you can reframe your beliefs so they align with your desires, and this is exactly what we did with Trudy. Here are Trudy's new and empowering beliefs that served her intentions and created new results.

- Even though I have been overweight most of my life, this is a brand-new moment in time and I'm trying something new, so I'll likely get new results.
- I find it easy to exercise outside my sessions with Michelle. I wake up early and exercise before work.
- Sugar is a poison that harms my body and is no good for me. Through regular meditation and relaxation, I perform well at work and have all the time I need to get everything done.
- I am calm and peaceful and everything is happening as it should.
- I am the only one responsible for my health and happiness, and my husband is the only one responsible for his. I can choose what I want to eat. Nobody can make me eat anything.
- My healthy is a priority because I am a priority. I deserve to be in a fit and healthy body I love.
- I enjoy spending time with myself and learning more about what motivates my actions.

- I am loved, safe, and protected, and it's okay to express my true feelings.
- It is okay to say *no*. I don't need to give a reason.

Two weeks later Trudy had dropped nine pounds of fat. I hugged her with glee and admiration. "See how powerful you are?" I said. "Congratulations on recognizing your innate abilities to change the beliefs that no longer serve you!"

If you develop the absolute sense of certainty that powerful beliefs provide, then you can get yourself to accomplish virtually anything, including those things that other people are certain are impossible.

Tony Robbins

Reframing Your Beliefs

Reframing is a powerful way to shift our old, limited perceptions to new, more empowering perceptions that we can accept as true, and thus expand the possibilities available to us in our lives. Once we formulated a new set of beliefs for Trudy, she then read these beliefs on a daily basis and began to *act as if* they were true even though at first she was not totally certain. After we added some energy work and emotional work to release her old beliefs from her nervous system, her behaviors and results changed.

When you believe you can—you will!

Exploring her current beliefs based on her internal mental software and then reframing those beliefs made it easier for Trudy to change her behaviors and experience new results. The previous beliefs she'd had about food, time, her husband, and herself produced a limiting reality for Trudy, which meant a limiting experience of life. Trudy was amazed at how powerful the practice of changing her beliefs really was. When Trudy changed her beliefs, her entire world changed, and it became easier and easier to find the time necessary to eat well and exercise regularly.

Change the way you look at things and the things you look at change.

Dr. Wayne Dyer

The Power of Belief

A belief can be either a mental roadblock that prevents you from experiencing what you want or the doorway to everything you want. We can use a belief to maintain "things as they are," or we can consciously adapt our beliefs to what best serves our intentions.

It is exciting to realize that we now have a tremendous evolutionary advantage that gives us the conscious ability to direct our outcomes on an individual and collective level. We get to *choose* how we want to experience life and choose the beliefs that support what we wish to accomplish.

Conversely, it also helps to recognize that, if we insist on holding onto disempowering beliefs simply to be consistent with our past, with society, or with our family and friends' beliefs, we will thwart our potential and live under a profound disadvantage.

I know people who have chosen to keep certain beliefs because they were familiar and it was comfortable to do so. Even if they didn't like the results they were producing and experiencing in life, the consistency between their beliefs and their experiences at least confirmed that their worldview was the "correct one," in spite of the misery it caused them.

We are each responsible for the quality of our lives—part of this responsibility involves choosing what we want to believe.

Are Your Beliefs Making You Fat?

In his book, *The Biology of Belief,* eminent scientist Bruce Lipton, PhD, writes that ". . . the fundamental behaviors, beliefs, and attitudes we observe in our parents become 'hard-wired' as synaptic pathways in our subconscious minds during childhood. Once programmed into the subconscious mind, they control our biology for the rest of our lives . . . or at least until we make the effort to reprogram them."[1] He explains that children, until the age of about six, have the same brainwave frequency as someone who has been put into a state of hypnosis and therefore are in a highly "suggestible, programmable state."[2] He goes on to say that "This gives us an important clue as to how children . . . can download the incredible volume of information they need to thrive in their environment . . . Young children carefully observe their environment and download the worldly wisdom offered by parents directly into their subconscious memory. As a result, their parents' behaviors and beliefs become their own."[3]

Are we really living our own lives, or the lives of
our parents and their parents and their parents . . . ?

Lipton gives an example of how limiting beliefs might be transferred by a parent to a child, who then unconsciously adopts them as his or her own: "Given the precision of [a young child's] behavior-recording system, imagine the consequences of hearing your parents say you are a 'stupid child,' or 'You do not deserve to have what you want' or 'You will never amount to anything' . . . or 'You will always be fat because you're so lazy.'"[4]

Any and all information we take in as children is downloaded into the subconscious memory as absolute facts, just as surely as bits and bytes are downloaded into the hard drive of your computer. During early development, the child's consciousness has not evolved enough to critically assess what is truth or not or what is going to serve them the best in their life. The child simply accepts what they're downloading without question.

Then the day comes when what we believe doesn't match what we want or what we feel is our truth inside.

For many of my clients, the idea that we can *choose* beliefs seems radical—at first. We assume that we believe what is true and that we are right about everything we believe. If someone disagrees with us, we assume they are wrong. People will do anything to maintain their beliefs. In some instances people are even willing to *kill* and *die* for them.

But a belief is just a thought and an assumption. Some beliefs may be based on "facts" more than others, but if you have ever taken a good look at the fields of social science such as government ideology and policy, history, and anthropology, or even the "harder" sciences such as medicine, astronomy, and physics, you know that what we call "truth" is changing all the time. Our description of truth—i.e., our beliefs—has always been subjective. So if rigid disciplines such as medicine and physics can change their beliefs regularly, why shouldn't we, as long as they reflect the deeper truth we're learning—like the fact that we deserve to live in a fit, healthy body we love? What better reason is needed to encourage you to take on some healthier, more empowering beliefs?

> To believe in the things you can see and touch is no belief at all. But to believe in the unseen is both a triumph and a blessing.
>
> Bob Proctor

The Placebo Effect Proves the Power of Belief

Steve Bavister and Amanda Vickers point out in their book, *Teach Yourself NLP*, that: "There's considerable evidence for the power of beliefs across a range of fields, but the Placebo Effect is probably the most compelling. Research has shown time and again that a significant proportion of patients who are given placebos believe them to be therapeutic and actually get well. In one study, patients were separated into two groups, all of which required a procedure for angina, chest pains that can lead to heart attacks. All were anaesthetized in the normal way, but just one of the groups actually underwent the operation. The members of the other group only had their skin cut, to make them *believe* the procedure had taken place. Those operated on showed a useful 40 percent improvement, while those who had the placebo surgery had an astonishing 80 percent recovery rate. Such studies show clearly that our beliefs can determine the way things turn out. They're not mere 'thoughts,' they're instructions. Believing something sends a psycho-neurological message through your entire mind/body system that seeks to make it happen."

Belief consists in accepting the affirmation of the soul; unbelief, in denying them.

Ralph Waldo Emerson

I don't intend to imply anything about whether any specific beliefs are objectively true or false. For example, I know what I believe, but due to the subjective nature of belief described above, I would never want to push my beliefs on someone else. The important point in the context of health and weight loss is that there are as many different worldviews as there are people, and thankfully, through new insights in the field of physics, we now understand that our beliefs create our reality, for better or worse, and that we have the power to change our beliefs and thus change our reality for the better.

THOUGHT PROVOKERS

- *What do you believe about your body?*
- *What do you believe about your capabilities to transform your body and your health?*
- *What do you believe about food?*
- *What do you believe about sugar?*
- *Do you believe you have all the time you need to achieve the health and body you want?*
- *What do you believe about time?*

- *Do you believe you have the support you need?*
- *What are your beliefs about health, family, money, religion, spirituality, yourself?*

Beliefs Are the Illusions through Which We Experience the World

According to the laws of physics, when we look at the world through our unique set of filters and illusions (our beliefs), the world can only project back to us what we already believe. In his book, *The Power of Awareness*, Neville Goddard cites the experiments in visual perception that scientists Merle Lawrence and Adelbert Ames Jr. conducted at the Dartmouth psychology laboratory. Based on their experiments, they concluded that: "what you see when you look at something *depends not so much on what is there as on the assumption you make when you look*. Since what we believe to be the 'real' physical world is actually only an 'assumptive' world, it is not surprising that these experiments prove that what appears to be solid reality is actually the result of expectations or assumptions. Your assumptions [beliefs] determine not only what you see, but also what you do, for they govern all your conscious and subconscious movements towards the fulfillment of themselves."[5]

Are you living your life at the cause or effect of your beliefs?

Is it possible that the very nature of our experience of reality is based only on what we believe or assume it to be? Yes! The science of belief sounds almost fantastical, like a sci-fi novel describing a possible future or universe where humans can create anything they want simply by believing it to be so. But consider this latest conundrum in the study of genetics before you determine how far-fetched this fantasy might be.

Geneticists have traditionally looked to DNA as the determining factor of our "destiny." It was, and still is, believed by many that we each contain within our body a kind of code that dates back to our family and family's families that can tell the story of our likely future. This field of science looks at our predispositions for certain health conditions and behaviors based on the biology passed down through generations. The idea then is that we not only get our family patterns through socialization, we also take on our ancestors' encoded biology, including body type. What geneticists have proposed is that our DNA tells our story even before we do. And we can look to our encoded destiny to unravel the inevitability of our physical and even psychological conditions and lives.

This is an interesting dilemma. On one hand, those who have never been able to lose weight could quite easily buy into the idea that "my weight is not my fault." Then if they *believe* they can't lose weight because it's their genetic destiny, they won't lose weight and will possibly give up any attempts to do so. They stop attempting to lose weight because now they hold a very powerful belief—scientifically "proven" to be true—that runs counter to what they want. Or they could choose to believe that they *can* be fit *regardless* of the fact that their grandmother and great-grandmothers before them were fat. Fortunately, more recent studies support the latter—it is now a new scientific fact that our DNA can be, and is, literally altered by our beliefs.

You Can Change Your DNA through Belief

There is now new research supported by Bruce Lipton, PhD, who states in *The Biology of Belief* that: ". . . the new science of *Epigenetics*, which literally means 'control above the genes,' has completely upended our conventional understanding of genetic control. Epigenetics is the science of how environmental signals select, modify, and regulate gene activity."[6] In *The Spontaneous Healing of Belief*, scientist, spiritual teacher, and author Gregg Braden cites research from the late 1990s and early 2000s that proves: "Human belief (and the feelings and emotions surrounding it) directly changes [our] DNA. . . Our beliefs hold all of the power we need for all of the change we choose: the power to send healing commands to our immune systems, stem cells, and DNA . . . to heal our deepest hurts, breathe life into our greatest joys, and literally create our everyday Reality. Through our beliefs we hold the gift of the single most powerful force in the universe: the ability to *change our lives, our bodies, and our world by choice*" (emphasis mine).[7]

This new awareness reveals that the activity of our genes is constantly being modified in response to life experiences, which again emphasizes that our perceptions of life shape our biology, and not the other way round.

This is a stunning reversal of what we have always believed about DNA—that it carries forth our genetic story. In short, you can change your DNA by changing your beliefs!

> By forming beliefs that affirm what is possible and telling better stories about what we are capable of, we use the gift of personal choice to create for ourselves a new reality.

My own experience working with clients every day on their health and body issues also proves this newly discovered fact. While family history would seem to predict that losing weight was once impossible, we can now have the body we choose because we *believe* we can, and because we intentionally decide that for ourselves. Clients in my wellness facility are proving so all the time. Take Sarah as an example of what belief can do.

Sarah's Story

I once worked with a 54-year-old client named Sarah. When Sarah came to see me, she had over 100 extra pounds to lose. One of her biggest challenges with her weight was controlling her portions and managing to regularly fuel her body throughout the day. Sarah would often eat almost nothing during the entire day, then gorge on an enormous meal at dinner time, sometimes consisting of three different courses. Sarah was very forthcoming with her beliefs around eating:

- Eating too frequently will cause me to gain weight, not lose it.
- Meal times are the *most* important time for families to be together.
- I would *never* make less than a three-course meal at dinner time. It's just not a part of my culture and not the way we do things. That would be rude!
- I spend so much time making these meals out of love, my family should eat everything I put in front of them, otherwise it's considered rude.
- Of course you need a dessert after dinner!
- Eating helps me relieve my boredom.

Can you see how these beliefs were perpetuating Sarah's challenge with her weight? But once we reframed Sarah's beliefs just like we did for Trudy, Sarah began experiencing different results. Sarah not only modified her old eating habits, she began losing a lot of weight. And the best part for her was knowing that she was instilling healthier habits in her children and her family. She stopped insisting everyone finish everything on their plates and started eating smaller, more frequent meals throughout the day so she wouldn't be so ravenous by dinner time. She also stopped serving dessert.

> *Your beliefs become your thoughts. Your thoughts become your words. Your words become your actions. Your actions become your habits. Your habits become your values. Your values become your destiny.*
> Mahatma Gandhi

Think of Beliefs Like This

Here's what the scientific research cited above practically means. Think of your mind as the hard drive or storage medium of a computer and your DNA as the operating system or master control system. Then imagine that your most empowering beliefs—both unconsciously preinstalled and consciously chosen and downloaded—comprise the current software program. You may not understand how it works, but you can actually see what commands it has programmed into it by the results you are producing in your life. For example, if you have always found it extremely challenging to stop eating your way through a packet of Skittles when you are stressed out, even though it makes life worse for you when you do, then your software needs to be upgraded and your mental hardware cleared of all viruses.

Now think of your unconscious, limiting beliefs as stealth viruses, often intractable and hidden from view. Though you cannot see them, they wrest control of the overall functioning of the computer no matter what commands you type on the keyboard. When your computer is infected with a virus, it is not unlike the mind when it is operating from a set of limiting beliefs that have been downloaded without your awareness. It won't listen to what you want it to do. The system is operating on automatic, obeying unconscious commands far beyond your control.

To change your mental programming, you have to gain command over the whole system and banish the commands that run counter to the new software. You need to open up the computer and see what's going on in there—which is what we do when we *go within* and self-inquire about our beliefs. This is how you get the information you need to fix the problem.

Believing precedes achieving.

What We Believe Will Prove True for Us

What we believe in our heart absolutely determines our results and experiences in life. The following question is an excellent question to be asking yourself right now:

> *What do I need to believe about myself, my time, and/or my health in order to make my weight and health goals my reality tomorrow?*

If you believe something is possible, you *can* create it and achieve it. Great inventors, artists, and athletes are able to do extraordinary things because they chose to *believe* that what they wanted to invent or create or achieve was possible. And here is the second step in the process—they then *looked* for their beliefs to show up as true until they actually became true. Amazing, when you think about it deeply.

And now consider this also—how often do we *look* for what we *don't* want to be true? How many times do we step on the scale as unbelievers, waiting to see failure at every turn? How many times do we pull on our pants and expect them to be tight and uncomfortable? How many times do we begin a new diet and expect it to fail in a few days? How many times do we look in the mirror and believe what we see is the extent of our life? And isn't it true that you are then surprised when you experience something different than you believed? Don't you then question it? Don't you say something to yourself like, *"Oh well, this probably won't last, or it was just a fluke or coincidence"*? Come on, admit it.

THOUGHT PROVOKERS

- *Do your current beliefs really serve and benefit you?*
- *Do you believe you have the power to transform your body and change your life?*
- *Do you believe your body is capable of such transformation?*
- *Do you believe you deserve to be fit and healthy?*
- *Do you believe in yourself?*
- *Do you believe your weight issues are genetic?*
- *Do you believe you don't have time to take care of your body?*
- *Have you said it's too expensive to join a gym, hire a trainer, go to yoga classes, or buy organic food?*
- *Do you feel unlovable and unattractive because you are a large person?*
- *Do you believe life is better if you are thin?*
- *Do you believe you're sensual and sexy?*

- *If you are a mom, do you believe you have no time for yourself?*
- *Do you believe you need to count calories in order to shed unwanted pounds?*
- *Do you believe certain foods have power over you?*
- *Now ask yourself these questions:*
- *Where did my beliefs originate?*
- *How do I really know my beliefs are true?*
- *Am I willing to let go of the beliefs that do not serve me and my health?*
- *Who would I be free to be if I didn't believe the beliefs that are holding me back?*

New and Empowering Beliefs

I implore you to remember that if you believe something without a doubt, it *has* to show up as true for you. So if you want to live a certain kind of life, if you want to lose weight, if you want to be in a fabulous relationship, if you want to make more money and live your passions and your purpose, then start formulating beliefs right now that support these heart-felt desires. Get out your journal or flip to the journal pages at the end of this book and start writing down everything you want to believe that supports your intentions.

Listen to that voice inside your heart that speaks your truth and ask yourself: "What beliefs would be more empowering for me to have? What beliefs will allow me to achieve the outcomes and the body I want?" Then, like a scientist and inventor, go out in the world and look for evidence that these new and empowering beliefs are true. Allow these beliefs to show up as reality. As an example, when you choose to believe you "have all the time you need to eat right and exercise," you will notice this belief will prove true for you in your experience. You can even ask people who are living the life experiences you want, "What do you believe?" They take on their beliefs as your own.

All things are possible to those who believe.
Jesus Christ

Beliefs Can Heal the Sick

In his book *The Holographic Universe,* Michael Talbot puts it this way: "We act like addicts when someone tries to wrest from us the powerful opium of our dogmas."[8] And that is why it is not always easy to change our beliefs. You need to make a conscious choice and do the work of taking your mind down very different tracks. And you have very inspiring proof it works, even for those who are extremely physically sick.

Dr. Bernie S. Siegel, author of the book, *Love, Medicine, and Miracles,* found in his work with cancer patients that a shift in their beliefs could actually improve their health, and in many cases eliminate their illnesses altogether.[9] When you allow limiting beliefs to fall away and replace them with ones that support your highest intentions, you can literally create miracles. You don't have to figure it all out now. Just love yourself enough to try.

In my studio, when my clients tell me they aren't strong enough to lift heavy weights, I tell them I'm going to help them a bit (which is a teeny white lie, because I don't—instead I just rest my hands on the weights very lightly) and suddenly they have the strength to lift. What we believe is what we'll experience! Those in my studio who believe they are going to succeed always do. Those who do not, find they stumble and fall until we reframe what they believe to be possible.

Life-Affirming Beliefs

What we are today comes from our thoughts of yesterday, and our present thoughts build our life of tomorrow: Our life is the creation of our mind.
Buddha

Our spiritual leaders and sacred texts have said it over and over again, and quantum physics has proven it: when we believe something, that belief is fed back to us through our experiences. Quantum physics has shown us that not only do all vibrations attract similar vibrations, but the observer determines what he or she sees. Our most potent foundational beliefs (conscious and unconscious) determine what we see, which activates our thoughts and feelings, which then attract people and experiences who mirror back to us exactly what we believe on the deepest level. The goal is to make positively empowering beliefs such a habit that we do it unconsciously and consistently.

Awareness

The first step of course, is to become *aware* of the exact unconscious beliefs that currently undermine our confidence and sabotage our best intentions in each moment. This is why the concept and practice of awareness, covered in chapter 2, is so important. Even if we don't yet recognize these thoughts in the moment they occur, we can still easily uncover our strongly held beliefs by being aware of the experiences we have from day to day. From this awareness, we are then empowered to make changes in our belief systems, thoughts, emotional responses, and behavior in order to support, nurture, and create the bodies and lives we really want.

It is up to you to decide to believe in what you truly desire. Are you ready to expand your mind and limitless potential to encompass your wildest dreams?

Practice: Believing Is Seeing

Examine and Reframe Your Beliefs

Step 1: List your beliefs about the following in your personal journal or the journal pages in this book:

- Health
- Time
- Your capabilities and abilities
- Food
- Money

- Spirituality/religion
- Family
- Sex
- Relationships

Step 2: For each belief you identified, ask yourself the following questions:

- How do I know this belief is true?
- Where did this belief originate?
- Whose belief was this before I chose to claim it?
- Am I willing to let go of this belief?
- What feelings and emotions arise surrounding this belief?
- What do I make this belief mean about me?
- How has this belief come to define me and form my life stories?
- What could I choose to believe instead that's more empowering for me?
- What other beliefs might be attached to this belief that also need my examination?
- What feelings and emotions arise when I think about not believing this belief anymore?
- How are these beliefs intertwined with my stories and identity?
- Who would I be if I did not believe this belief to be true?
- Am I willing to entertain the idea of a new belief and see what arises as a result of intentionally looking for it in my experience? If not, why not?
- What resistances (beliefs), if any, arose for me during this practice?

Step 3: Against each belief you identify, write a new and empowering belief that supports your intentions and desires.

Step 4: Write any additional beliefs that will support your intentions. (Tip: Ask for the beliefs of someone you know who is already achieving the results and lifestyle you want.)

Step 5: Begin to *act as if* these beliefs are true for you in your life. Meditate on them daily, visualizing them as a reality in your life, and read through your list of new beliefs several times a day. You can also write them on sticky notes and stick them around your home and workplace. I also like to pray to have my beliefs show up in my experiences.

Step 6: If you find you struggle to embrace a new and empowering belief and release an old, fixed, and limiting belief, see chapter 4: you may need to *go within* and dig into the emotions that surround these beliefs so that you can begin releasing those emotional roadblocks. Finally, if this doesn't completely resolve the issue for you, find someone like myself to perform some additional emotional and energy work to completely remove your sabotaging beliefs from your nervous system and ultimately your life.

CHAPTER 4

MENTAL NOISE

Be not conformed to this world but be transformed
by the renewing of your mind.
Romans 12:2

love to walk. I enjoy exercising with weights, doing dance-fitness classes, and boxing, but when it comes to a mindful workout that also burns fat and is good for my health, walking is my go-to activity. Walking evokes a peace and tranquility in me, and I find it also stills and quiets my mind. When I walk, I fall into in a natural rhythm that becomes hypnotic and allows me to fully inhabit my body.

I live by a lake, which I'm absolutely thrilled about. I love the water. It naturally seems to open my heart and restore the feeling of oneness and peace in me. Water is my therapy—it's where I go to regain my center in life and am able to recall that all is happening as it should and there is nothing in life to fear.

Everyone needs a place like this—where they rest and feel centered, as though they are home.

One particular day, as I was out walking, I wasn't looking to reconnect to my center. My son and I had been inside most of the morning, doing our weekend chores, and cabin fever was setting in—which is to say we were beginning to get on each other's nerves. Outside time, with its wall-less space and fresh air, was exactly what we needed. We went outside and headed toward the lake, primarily because it has a terrific park that my son loves to play in. He was cycling ahead of me like a mad thing on his new three-wheel tricycle—a gift from my brother, who would've happily kept the trike for himself if he wasn't in his thirties and over six feet tall. Boys and their toys!

While walking along, feeling the warmth of the sun on my face and watching my little guy pedaling furiously up ahead in an attempt to break the latest speed record, I couldn't help but feel an overwhelming sense of gratitude for my life. I have a gorgeous and fabulous son, a beautiful home, family and friends who support and love me, a career that nourishes and feeds my soul, and I'd just had a medical examination that gave me a clean bill of health. I looked up at the sky, breathed with appreciation, and winked lovingly at God. Life is good, no doubt about it.

But my "aaahhh . . . life is good" moment was suddenly interrupted when I noticed something up ahead on the grass. I frowned with some disappointment—garbage. I am a stickler for litter and I wish people wouldn't treat the earth like a garbage can. As I got closer to the object in question, I realized it was an empty cigarette packet. As I bent down to pick it up, determined to put it in the garbage bin just a few feet away, I froze midway at the sight of the image leaping off the packaging. It was a photograph of the inside of someone's mouth—covered in sores and pus. A big, red warning notice screamed: "Smoking causes oral cancer; puff away at your own risk!"

In a nano-second, my Zen-like feelings of peaceful oneness and gratitude vanished and I became awash with intense fear. My attention and focus rushed out of my body like a speeding tsunami, and I wanted to turn and bolt and get as far away as possible from this frightening and hideous image.

Instead, I stood there like a drugged zombie, while the following nonsense unfolded in my head:

Oh my God! That could be your mouth on that box! You used to smoke, Michelle! Remember? REMEMBER? You should never have smoked! What were you thinking?! Oh my God, I don't want cancer! I just lost three friends to cancer last year! And they were so young—and such good people. I'm a good person too! Oh my goodness—my son! I can't die now! Who will look after my little boy?

Michelle, get a grip. Focus! You're not dead! You're right here, and your son still has his mother—calm down. Yeah, but my friends' children don't have their parents anymore. They were such amazing people! Stop thinking this way! Why are you thinking this way? You're going to create this! You are going to manifest cancer! Stop it! Breathe . . . Remember, your thoughts are things—thoughts are things . . . Is that a man's or a woman's mouth? What does that matter? Man or woman, it's a terrible thing for anyone to have to endure! I will pray for this person. Poor fellow—there I go again! Calm down! Remember, everything happens for a reason, Michelle. Oh yeah, breathe . . . just relaaaaax.

Why am I still looking at this image? What if this happens to me? How much did I used to smoke? I need to think . . . two a day? Six a day? No, wait. It wasn't that many . . . how many was it now? Not that many—but you did smoke, Michelle! Yes, I know that, but I was just a social smoker! There's a difference! How many cigarettes would one need to smoke to get oral cancer? Need to check that one with Mr. Google. Wait! Did I turn off the computer this morning? Need to send Mum an e-mail. Looks like a man's mouth. Maybe mouth cancer only happens to males. What? This is ridiculous.

WHY ARE YOU STILL LOOKING AT THE PICTURE? Walk away. That's it . . . You can do it . . . Walk aw—Did I take the eggs off the stove? Mmm . . . I need some water. My mouth is itchy. I should've brought some water . . . I'm hungry. You're not hungry; you're scared. Damn right, I'm scared. I don't want cancer. Stop it! You're not getting cancer. Go eat a burger . . . A burger? I don't want a burger. I feel like a salad . . . with chicken . . . and . . . Okay, STOP! That's it! My mind has taken over. Time to focus on the fear that's fueling these ridiculous thoughts. What am I really afraid of here and . . . Where did my kid go?!

At this point I suddenly realized I had not seen my child for what was probably only a millisecond, but it felt like an eternity while I pumped out automatic thoughts like a machine gun. Frantically, I tore my eyes away from the cigarette box to see my son rapidly approaching the roadside and I was certain he wouldn't be able to stop, regardless of how much tread his new shoes had on them. I envisioned him flying out on to the road and being flattened by a car, with me running toward him like a lunatic, screaming and crying, awash with grief and the regret of not telling him how much I love him—even though I had actually told him at least eighty-two times already that day.

Then I stopped and became aware of what was *really* happening: my son was cycling safely ahead of me, and there was a small cardboard box with a picture of an infected mouth lying on the ground. That's it. That's all there was. Everything else, the nonsense in my head, the thoughts and the feelings, were not a true reflection of what was *actually* happening. But they were a reflection of my internal processes, which were being fueled by feelings of fear in that moment. When I became aware of my internal experience and acknowledged the fear that was fueling it, I could then cease participating in all the mental nonsense associated with the fear. This is the power of awareness. The ability to observe what we are thinking, feeling and experiencing on the inside, while remaining present and aware of what is happening on the outside.

Disempowering Noise

In a single day, the average person experiences an estimated 50,000-70,000 thoughts per day. Of these thoughts, it is postulated that 70–80 percent of these thoughts are limiting and disempowering. Even more disturbing is that the majority of our thoughts are total nonsense and direct our attention to either worry about a future that hasn't even happened yet or dwell on a past that has gone and cannot be changed. Then, to add even further injury to this insane reality, we then *believe* this mental nonsense and identify the truth of who we are, our capabilities, and potential with these baseless, limiting, and disempowering thoughts. We hear these thoughts and we say, *Yeah, that's right. I am a total idiot for missing my exercise session today. I am lazy, and everybody is looking at my fat stomach.* Nonsense!

Meanwhile, while life is occurring in the moment—and in divine perfection, I might add—we are missing it completely, because we are focused not on the present but on the thoughts inside our head that are complete and utter fantasy and not the truth of reality at all. Those of you who meditate regularly (and I hope that many of you do) will likely be more aware of this tendency, since when we meditate deeply, we move from being *attached* to our thoughts to *observing* our thoughts instead. We don't *identify* with what we are thinking; we are simply *aware* of what we are thinking.

Then, from this place of awareness and observation, we can easily see what a total car wreck our mental activity really is. We can *see* our thoughts from the place of awareness and we can objectively decide whether we want to entertain thoughts like: *I don't have time,* or *Why did I choose to wear this outfit today? I look awful!* Then, through the power and intention of our heartfelt awareness and desires, we can choose not to entertain any of these thoughts at all. Instead we choose to focus on the space *between* the words of our thoughts and the silence in which our thoughts rise and fall.

You Are Not What You Think

When I first tell people that what they think isn't true and that their thoughts have no bearing whatsoever on who think they are, they look at me like I should be wearing a straitjacket. They often say something like, "What do you mean my thoughts aren't true?" or "I don't understand you when you say 'my thoughts are not true and not who I am.' Of course they are! They're coming out of my head, aren't they?!" My response to this question, which can arouse fear and uncertainty, is yes . . . and *no.* Yes, you are experiencing the thoughts arising from within your head (via awareness), but no, they are not *your* thoughts, and no, they do not determine who you are. But they are responsible right now for the results you're experiencing because you *believe* that they are true and because you are giving them your attention by focusing on them.

Thoughts are things—energetic frequencies that arise out of nothingness and go back into nothingness. Like a kite in flight, a thought will fly right by you unless you reach up and grab it, and then claim it as your own.

Our thoughts can come from a variety of sources. Sometimes they come from our beliefs—for example, if we believe that we are not coordinated, when an opportunity to sign up for a fitness dance class comes up, we think: *I can't sign up for that class—I'd embarrass myself.* Sometimes our thoughts are triggered by a current sensory experience, such as a song or a picture or a smell that reminds us of a past experience. And sometimes they are utterly random and meaningless: *Why is a pickle called a pickle and not a pumpkin?*

Whatever their source, as we dwell on our thoughts, they trigger feelings (and vice versa), and then our feelings motivate our behavior. So when a thought rises into your awareness, and if you believe that this thought is not only real but part of you, then naturally you will listen to and believe this thought because that's what's you've always done. Moreover, when you pay attention to your thoughts, your attention gets distracted from the present moment—*this precise moment*—and now you're trapped in the world of your thoughts. Sometimes these thoughts can be pleasant and exciting, but most of the time they are debilitating and evoke feelings of fear, anxiety, panic, distrust, jealousy, resentment, and a host of other limiting emotional experiences.

How Thoughts Can Fuel Your Health and Weight Struggles

What you think about on a regular basis drives your motivation, influences your behaviors, and thus determines your results. Our thoughts can be very distracting and disempowering, and if we let them take hold, they can destroy us. If you continue to entertain every one of your thoughts, believing that your thoughts are always true and real, you will constantly struggle to awaken your true potential and experience life as it *really* is, which is *unlimited possibility.* The thoughts you entertain and speak fuel the results you are experiencing within your body and your life.

What's in the Silence?

Beyond the noise of our thoughts lies the silence of our minds, which contains everything we have ever wanted to know and/or need to know. When we can disentangle ourselves from the noise in our heads and rest in this tranquil, alive, loving, and profoundly intelligent silence, we can *allow* that which we want to attract and experience in our lives to naturally and organically arise as an idea or suggestion. We may experience it as a thought, a *feeling*, or simply as a *knowing* that serves as a strong foundation for our intentions. But the point is that when we can rest in the silence, we can choose what thoughts to focus on, and thus what our reality will be.

If this information seems more than you can swallow, use this resistance and/or confusion to recognize right now, in this very moment, that this resistance that is happening in your head is exactly what I'm talking about. You are having thoughts and these thoughts are telling you things and you are believing and/or entertaining these thoughts. If this information is very new to you then your brain is desperately trying to search for some reference point of currently held knowledge on which to hang the coat of this content on. Because a new idea pushes our mind to the boundary conditions of its awareness, for a few moments this process can feel like confusion, frustration, fear or even panic. Yet what precedes an 'aha' moment is total and utter confusion which means, *you are exactly where you're meant to be right now* and everything you're experiencing is perfect. Any moment now you are going to have a breakthrough!

Experience Is the Best Teacher

The best way to get a firm grasp on what is being shared in this chapter is to experience it firsthand, as opposed to attempting to understand it intellectually. While many will say that knowledge is power, it's also true that if you think you've figured it all out, you can be certain you haven't. To experience the power and wisdom that arises from observing our thoughts instead of *becoming* our thoughts, the best practice is through Awareness Meditation™, which you will learn how to do at the end of this chapter.

However, the key to connecting and becoming one with the silence in our minds is heartfelt awareness and attention. So in addition to meditation, we can also quiet our minds when we *move* our body, as in exercise, dance, and yoga. The reason is that as we move physically, our attention *moves away* from the noise (thoughts) in our head to the aliveness and activity occurring within our bodies. For example, when we engage in activities like boxing and martial arts, there often isn't time to think, because we need to be present to what's happening in the moment; if we don't pay attention, we're likely going to get hit or kicked. Similarly, when we lift heavy weights, or in dance and yoga, the choreography of the movement requires us to *pay attention* to our bodies; sometimes different body parts turn, in order to *move* our bodies in a specific and particular way. Therefore, as we more fully inhabit our bodies, we pay less attention to our "heads."

The true magic happens as you continue to practice these movements. Soon you'll find you don't even need to focus on your body anymore, as the energy of life's flow will naturally arise from within you and move with the natural flow of life around you. Imagine a leaf when the wind collects it from the ground and gathers it up high into the air. The leaf becomes *at one* with the wind, and it goes wherever the wind carries it. When we move our attention out of thought and instead into this flow of life (or what many are now calling "intention"), then you'll find that you don't have to *think* so much about anything anymore, because life will naturally lead you exactly where you want to go.

THOUGHT PROVOKERS

- *What thoughts are running through your head right now?*
- *Where are these thoughts arising from?*
- *Can you isolate their source within your body?*

- *Do you hear, feel, taste, smell, or see your thoughts (or all of these)?*
- *Can you discern between thoughts that are just thoughts, and the thoughts that are also beliefs?*
- *When you focus on your thoughts, how are they making you feel?*
- *What were you thinking about right before you started thinking about what you were thinking about?* ☺
- *Have you ever noticed the silence between your words and thoughts?*
- *What would it feel like not to think at all?*

Sandra's Story

I once coached a woman named Sandra who suffered intensely from anxiety and panic attacks. One minute she'd be happy as anything, without a care in the world. The next she'd be breaking out in a facial heat rash and finding it difficult to breathe. Her muscles would tighten and her hands would clench into white-knuckling fists. Her chin would drop, her jaw would lock, and she'd feel as though she was about to faint.

Instead of going outside for answers, I invited Sandra to go within and invite me into her mental and emotional world. I invited her to describe for me in intimate detail what she was feeling, picturing inside her mind, sensing what thoughts she was choosing to listen to and become, and to describe her experience as best she could sequentially, from the moment she was feeling good to the point where everything changed and she felt panicked.

Without going into every detail of Sandra's experience, we discovered some specific thoughts that manifested in Sandra's body physiologically when she chose to focus on them. These included thoughts like: *What if I have a car accident on the way to work? What if the plane crashes, and as we are hurtling toward the ground my head snaps off and then my headless body ends up floating in the ocean and I get eaten by sharks? Who will look after my kids? What if I choke on this piece of chicken I'm eating and there is nobody around to perform the Heimlich maneuver and I'm left to die here alone and in pain?* Finally, *I can't breathe, I can't breathe! Oh my God, I can't breathe!*

Truth or Fiction?

Now you may be reading these thoughts of Sandra's and think: *Wow, I'd never think those thoughts—that's nutty,* or *Oh my God, that poor woman,* or *Yes, I can relate—this happens to me also.* Whatever your thought response was, that's all it was—a thought. We've all had these crazy thoughts, and our thoughts can only make *us* crazy if we let them.

In Sandra's experience, these types of thoughts felt very real and intensely frightening, as you can imagine. Sandra really did believe that she would likely have some tragic accident, die, and not be able to breathe. It was as though Sandra was watching a horror movie, and at some point during the movie, she thought she was *in* the movie and not *watching* it. Over time, the repetition of these thoughts and her physiological responses became linked neurologically, and finally, regardless of what was happening in the world around her, just one of those thoughts would trigger an overwhelming state of panic and fear, whereas two seconds ago she'd felt safe and calm.

To assist Sandra with her anxiety, I needed her to 1) realize her thoughts were not real, 2) create a neurological interruption in her nervous system so her body stopped responding with a fearful flight response to certain thoughts, images, and/or sensations, and 3) begin the practice of meditation, so she could begin to observe her thoughts without entertaining them. When Sandra began to realize her thoughts had no power in and of themselves, but only the power she gave them by entertaining them with her attention, her thoughts began losing their power. When we cease giving our thoughts our power and attention, they eventually get snuffed out like a candle in the rain. The more Sandra gave her attention and power to the *silence* between her thoughts instead of to her thoughts themselves, the more relaxed and at peace she began to feel, and the less often her anxiety-producing thoughts seemed to occur.

After addressing and then releasing the root-cause beliefs and emotional blocks associated with many of Sandra's anxieties, such as her fear of dying, the less influence external triggers had—like riding in an airplane. Rooted in the silence in her mind, life began to feel as though it was significantly slowing down in a beautiful way for Sandra. She became much more aware of the present moment and the joy and peacefulness stillness brings. What used to stress and worry Sandra no longer seemed to faze her as much, and she found she was much more productive and produced better results when she focused on the stillness and not the mental noise. She also was able to stop binge-eating . . .

How Does This Apply to You?

What we think we become. And what we think we are, *we are*. Our thoughts can trigger our emotional states, which can direct our behaviors and determine our results. In other words, the thoughts you choose to entertain and *identify with* in large part explain why you're overweight.

Before you toss this book aside and throw a lit match on it, first pause for a second and ask yourself: *Who would I be if I didn't think the thoughts I do, and what new results may arise in my life and body if I experienced my thoughts very differently?* Ask yourself whether the thoughts in your head support your desires to be healthy, or keep you fat and overweight? Do you often think: *I don't have time to exercise today,* or *exercising is hard and difficult?* What about: *I'm too tired, I'll exercise tomorrow,* or *This one piece of cake won't hurt?* Do you recognize these thoughts, and do you give them your attention and power? Hopefully you've put that burning match out, and you're nodding your head, *Yes, I do!*

THOUGHT PROVOKERS

- *What thoughts do you have on a regular basis?*
- *How many of these thoughts impact your health and weight?*
- *What do you do as a result of these thoughts?*
- *How are these results working for you?*

The Thoughts We Entertain and the Words We Speak Matter

Proverbs 4:22 says, "Be careful how you think; your life is shaped by your thoughts." Internationally acclaimed author Eckhart Tolle says, "The primary cause of unhappiness is never the situation but your thoughts about it."[10] He also says—and I wholeheartedly agree—that "All true artists, whether they know it or not, create from a place of no-mind, from inner stillness."[11]

From my many years of experience as a transformation specialist, coach, trainer and healer working with hundreds of men and women around the world, and through my own personal journey and evolution, I am now convinced that true transformation can *only* arise from the place of inner stillness, and that our thoughts only get in the way.

If you repeatedly entertain thoughts like: *I am the fit fat girl,* or *I can't do a push-up,* then this will be your experience in life. I often tell my clients in the studio, if you want to *change* the way other people view you, change the way you view yourself—through your thinking. If you tell yourself you are weak, no good at squats, or are forever prone to injuries, this will directly affect your body's performance. You *will* be weak, no good at squats, and prone to repetitive injury. Your body hears every thought you entertain, takes it as a kind of command, and then functions, or dysfunctions, accordingly. If you allow thoughts like, *I am not coordinated, I can't do push-ups,* and *my back is weak and always has been,* then you are building roadblocks to your own desires.

Our Body Never Lies

All that we are is the result of what we have thought. The mind is everything. What we think, we become.
Maharishi Mahesh Yogi

Just as our thoughts dictate our experiences, they also impact our physical bodies. Numerous scientific and medical studies and years of personal clinical experience clearly prove that our bodies respond to the messages we repeatedly give it. As mentioned previously, what we believe about ourselves fuels our repetitive thoughts. In her books, *Heal Your Body* and *Heal Your Life,* thought pioneer Louise Hay explains how specific thought patterns create specific physical dysfunctions and diseases within the body. Hay personally overcame her battle with vaginal cancer by weeding out negative thoughts and replacing them instead with positive thoughts, which are like a healthy medicine for the body and soul. By the way, what I said earlier about remembering that we are not our thoughts applies to positive thoughts as well as negative ones. If you have a positive thought and it makes you feel good, then there's nothing wrong with entertaining this thought so long as you remember that you're *not* the thought. Otherwise you'll develop an addiction and attachment to that emotional response of *that* thought and then when another thought arises if the emotional response is not what you want, you'll attempt anything (like eating) to try bring it back. The key is not to permanently stay in one emotional state but to instead participate in the ride of what simply arises in the moment. Just like watching a movie in the cinema, you undergo a ton of different emotional experiences in just a few hours. But isn't that why you bought the ticket? Isn't the reason you are watching the movie for this exact reason?

Hay states in *Heal Your Body* that, "The point of power is right here and right now in our own mind. It doesn't matter how long we have had negative patterns, an illness, a rotten relationship, a lack of finances, or self-hatred; we can begin to make a change today. The thoughts we have held and the words we have repeatedly used have created our life and experiences up to this point."[12]

I can also personally attest to this truth. I overcame my battle with depression and anxiety simply by "changing my mind"—by altering my thoughts, beliefs, and perceptions. So if our thoughts and language are powerful enough to heal physical and emotional illness, what do you think *your* thoughts are doing to *your* body?

And remember, your words are powerful, too! Instead of saying, "I can't do a push-up," or "I can't hold a plank past twenty seconds," say to yourself the opposite, and see what happens. Say, "I *can* do a push-up and I *can* hold a plank for thirty seconds!" Feel how it alters your body's experience.

At first your body may not respond right away to new messages. This is only because it has become so conditioned to responding to all the negative messages you've been entertaining for years. But that's okay, because you're now discovering that you have the power to change what doesn't vbenefit you.

We are disturbed not by what happens to us, but by our thoughts about what happens to us.
Epictetus

The Power of Consciousness

It is said that energy flows where attention goes. Think of all the negative attention you pay your body. Just as I did as a teenage girl, too many people who come to my gym are being God-awful to their bodies with all their horrible feedback. The unconscious messages we dump in our body results in a distorted, unhappy self because the body is gullible and believes it all!

At the same time, we pay very little attention to the inside of the body—all the functions that are performed moment to moment that keep us alive! We deprive the body of the attention and appreciation it deserves.

Anyone can alter their experiences. Every individual can direct his or her consciousness (thought) to create and dramatically alter the reality he or she occupies. We each have this same generative ability. The only difference is that some are aware of it while others are not.

Those who remain unaware usually feel the "effects" of life, or that life happens *to them* rather than *with them*. But when these same people become aware of their innate power to experience a new reality, they suddenly recognize that we live in a conscious, evolving universe in which we each participate through our every thought and every action. They come to see that they can lead their mind and emotions, rather than being led *by* them. They use the powers of silence and stillness to guide their lives, and meditation is a regular practice. They make giant leaps in their awareness of life, and their life conditions therefore radically improve. This change is all based on a simple shift in their thinking—that their thoughts are *not who they are*, and they don't have to believe nor entertain the thoughts that arise in their awareness.

For forty years I have struggled with my weight and body image. I feel that I have tried just about every diet known to humankind. It is impossible to calculate exactly how much weight I have lost. I know that I have lost and gained over 300 lbs. I almost gave up hope until I met Michelle Armstrong and began applying the principles that she teaches. That was when my transformation towards an "Extraordinary Life" began.

I clearly recall my first private one-on-one personal training session with Michelle. I was afraid, nervous, and embarrassed about my physical state. Unlike an exercise class, I would not be able to hide in a corner and fake my fitness level. I wanted to be thinner and in better shape before I started working out. I felt vulnerable, but I knew my health and overall well-being were at risk. It was time for me to act.

I was embarking on a new journey and leaving my comfort zone. I didn't know it at the time, but Michelle would teach me a new mindset: a new way of thinking about myself, and a new approach to how to better care for myself and see myself. I had someone who believed in me!

In time, I also came to believe in myself and worked towards acquiring a healthy mind, body, and spirit. I now know that "I can do anything I want to do," "I am the source of my own comfort," and "Food is fuel and meets my nutritional needs." I had Post-it® notes all over my house saying, "I am 148 lbs."

While I am not at my end-goal weight yet, (although I have lost 70 pounds to date) something has fundamentally changed within me. In my mind I have already become 148 lbs., and it feels fantastic. Though the scale may not tell me I'm at my perfect weight yet, the fact that I am telling myself I am matters more than I ever thought it would! I'm happier, for one thing. Because this mindset I now have is a lot more motivating than always picturing myself as someone who still "has to" lose over one hundred pounds. As my image of myself changed, I began to think and act as a 148-pound woman.

For the first time in my entire life, I saw life and myself differently, and I loved what I saw. I see myself as a fit, trim, healthy, active, and confident woman. Anything is possible! I am honest with where I am, but I know what I believe is what I will become. The extra bags of weight I carry have become inconsequential. I consider the rest of the fat now as a temporary situation. I now know with certainty these extra bags of weight will soon be dropped.

Marianne

Your outer reality reflects your inner reality.

When you become aware that infinite possibilities exist out there in that subjective substance called "reality," for you to shape as you will, life becomes much more fun, exciting, and meaningful. When you realize that you are not limited by the boundaries of your thoughts and beliefs, your mind begins to transcend itself and you transform. Now it's no longer a matter of trying to muster the willpower to eat better and exercise regularly; now you genuinely desire to support your life force and vitality in the best ways possible!

You don't allow spontaneous thoughts to tell you untruths about yourself or your reality anymore. You can now choose new and greater possibilities for yourself. Simply start by expanding your mind beyond its usual, limited view of reality.

The following practices are designed to bring more awareness and insight into the manifestation of your thoughts, and how these thoughts are affecting your current experience and challenges with your weight. There is no right way or wrong to do these practices. There is no test you need to pass, nor can you fail at these practices. All that's required is the heartfelt desire to learn more about yourself, so you can lose the unhealthy weight you want to lose and live the life you want. Awareness is the first step to transformation. Engaging in these practices on a regular basis is going to give you that awareness. You can do it! I know you can . . .

Practices: Mental Noise

Awareness Meditation™

To begin to shift from *identifying with* thought to *observing* thought, engage in a daily practice of meditation as follows.

Find somewhere quiet where you will not be interrupted for ten to fifteen minutes, and sit with an erect spine and close your eyes. You may also lie down if it's more comfortable for your body, but it's best to sit if you can so your body doesn't think it's going to sleep. Then, with your eyes closed, draw your attention inward and begin focusing on your breathing. You don't need to alter your breathing; just observe it. After a minute or so of observing your breath, draw your attention to your body and just notice both the aliveness within you and any possible tension or stress that may be occurring within these areas.

Begin with your toes and feet. Work your way up your legs into your calves, your knees, your thighs, and your hips. Draw your attention to your abdomen, your chest, your shoulders, your arms, your hands, and your fingers. Finally, draw your attention to your neck, your face, your ears, and your scalp. As you observe each of these parts of your body, imagine breathing a white light of wellness and healing energy into these areas. If tension or stress is present, imagine you can wrap the tension in the light, pull it into your breath, and then allow it to exit your body each time you exhale.

Then, when all tension has been removed, draw your attention and awareness to your *thoughts*. Just as you can sit beside a busy highway and watch cars —of all different shapes, colors, models, and makes—drive by without feeling the need to get into each vehicle and allow it to take you wherever it is going without your choosing, do the same with your thoughts. Begin to see your thoughts as *things*—energetic things that are simply occurring with you as their witness. Notice each thought as it arises from the stillness and disappears back into the stillness. Notice that you do not need to attach yourself in any way to these thoughts. Notice that each thought has its own distinct characteristics and personality. Don't judge your thoughts, but be aware of their presence. You are merely the *observer*.

If, as you are observing your thoughts, a certain thought or series of thoughts evokes an emotion, be aware of the emotion as well without participating fully in it. Let your inner awareness and intuition share with you any insights about these emotions later, once your meditation is over. If you find that certain thoughts and/or emotions pull your attention away from *observing* to *experiencing*, just take a deep breath, observe and notice the shift from observing to experiencing, and then gently pull your inner focus and attention back to the present moment.

Then, when you've finished your meditation, take three deep breaths of gratitude and open your eyes. Journal your experiences and insights. It can also be helpful to date your journal entries if you would like to track your progress.

Shine the Spotlight on Your Thoughts

For the next three days, carry your journal around with you, and every time you become aware of a thought, write it down. Don't edit or tweak the thought in any way. Write it exactly as you hear it in your mind. After three days, review your journal entries and look for themes and repetitive thoughts. Mentally hold these thoughts up against what you *want* to be experiencing in your life and what it is you *are* experiencing your life. Then, on a separate sheet of paper and/or in your journal, write out one hundred thoughts that are in total alignment with and support your desires. You don't have to write all one hundred in one sitting. Take as much time as you need. If you find you get stuck and cannot think of more thoughts, seek out someone you know who is achieving the results and experiences you wish to have and interview them about *their* thinking. When they share thoughts that inspire and motivate you, write them down.

Once you have your one hundred thoughts, post them all over your house and your workplace so you can see them daily. You can also record them with your own voice and listen to them on a regular basis. As you practice shining the spotlight on your thoughts over time, coupled with the above meditation practice, you will notice your old thoughts arising less and less and your new ones arising more and more, simply because you are giving these new thoughts your attention and focus, and because you are willing to entertain them as a possibility in your life. Eventually, your nervous system will be programmed to automatically play these thoughts to automatically respond to situations and stress with these thoughts.

CHAPTER 5

THE HEART OF THE MATTER

Emotions are the voices of our souls.
Listen in love, and know there's nothing to fear.

In this chapter, we're truly going to get down to the heart of the matter: the core reason why you're struggling with your weight, even though you intellectually know everything you're "supposed" to be doing to get healthy. To do so, we're going to have to address those deep, usually painful emotions you've been running from, perhaps all your life. You probably know which ones I'm talking about. You've ignored them, built walls around them, and wrapped those walls with barbed wire. But the truth is that even your best efforts can never really suppress these emotions. They're making themselves known right now, although you may not recognize them. The real reason for your struggles with weight is not poor diet, lack of exercise, or even genetics. If you are experiencing your life in an overweight or obese body, it is because you have suppressed your truest feelings and stopped *feeling* your emotional body. When you can liberate your emotions and set them free, the addictive habit of needing to eat (or not to eat) will dissolve.

Before we explore the depth of your emotional self, I want you to first know that it's okay to feel afraid of and resistant to exploring your feelings. Many people are afraid to look at their emotional world. But this resistance is a roadblock to your emotional liberation and thus to your liberation from weight struggles, and you must face it head on. As you will discover in this chapter, beneath this resistance lies the fear of vulnerability and rejection. This fear can manifest in the form of debilitating and limiting feelings of shame, but however it manifests, you will eventually need to *name* this fear and face it in order to heal and move forward.

I want to share with you a Facebook post shared by one of my clients, Tracy, who was participating in one of my group transformation programs. You'll have to excuse the language if it offends you, but it speaks the powerful truth of how Tracy really felt. I acknowledge and applaud Tracy for her courage in sharing her thoughts and feelings publicly. See if you can identify with any or all of what Tracy says. This is a gal who had suppressed a huge part of her emotional self because of the way she'd been raised.

I have spent the last couple days trying to decide if this transformation program is right for me or not. Last week's coaching session, where I was invited to share personal feelings, left me feeling very uncomfortable, embarrassed, sad, and upset. Sharing personal feelings and private thoughts is something I have difficulty with. In the environment I was raised, we were not encouraged to talk about our feelings or emotions; this was considered a sign of weakness. So I quickly learned to build a little bubble around me and keep my emotions to myself. Little did I know, this defense mechanism of mine had some debilitating side effects, one of which is my weight. As an adult, able to make my own decisions, I have difficulty sharing what I feel and standing up for myself. Then, when I do, I start to get upset at myself because deep down I know I have nothing to be ashamed about, but I just can't seem to get the feeling of shame off me. Then I start to feel sorry for myself, then I start to get mad, then I start to get embarrassed, then I start to eat. . . It's a huge cycle of crappy, annoying, confusing, fattening emotions. . .

"I signed up for this program to drop a few pounds and change my pant size. I didn't expect to drop a crap load of emotional baggage and change my mentality! If Michelle thinks she can fix my fifty shades of f***ed-up-ness, then I say, why not?"

Tracy

THOUGHT PROVOKERS

- *How were feelings managed when you were a child?*
- *Was it okay for you to express your true feelings?*
- *How did your parents manage their feelings?*
- *Was it okay to express sadness, hurt, anger, or fear?*

How Do I Know if I'm Suppressing My Feelings?

To put it bluntly, if you're overweight or obese and having body issues, you're suppressing your emotions. Eating more (or less) food than your body needs is not the true source of your weight problem. It is the *symptom* of suppressing the natural occurrence of emotions as they arise in the body—

and *this* is the cause that needs to be healed. When you disallow the truth of your emotional self to surface, you are ignoring and suppressing the voice of your soul and what needs to be conveyed from the heart. Your emotions are like beautiful signposts that bring your attention to something specific arising in the moment.

Clients will often say to me, "But I do get angry and I do get sad, so how is it that I'm suppressing my feelings?" Because the emotions that we *do* allow are often not what I like to call the "root cause" emotions, but rather the symptomatic feelings of these root-cause emotions. Our root-cause emotions are the heart of the matter—they are the emotions we don't want and are afraid to face. So yes, you may be feeling some of your emotions, but it's the root-cause emotions and feelings at the heart of the matter that you need to be aware of, and where you need to be directing your attention.

Here are some indicators of emotional avoidance and suppression:

- Difficulty talking about yourself with others
- A feeling of safety when eating and being by yourself
- A knot in the stomach that can't be identified
- Lack of interest in life, apathy, or a "who cares" attitude
- Explosive outbursts, rage, disgust, resentment
- Anxiety
- Inability to forgive
- Feelings of helplessness and hopelessness
- Boredom
- Putting on a happy face when you feel angry, resentful, or depressed inside
- A deep sense of separation and aloneness
- Fear of vulnerability and unrelenting feelings of shame and guilt
- Disconnection and distance from the world around you
- Inability to experience joy, difficulty laughing, loss of sense of humor
- Feeling overly judgmental, angry, or envious towards others

- Comparing yourself to others
- Agitation and discomfort in a room full of people and family
- Low self-esteem
- Numbness
- Lack of confidence
- Feelings of abandonment
- Intense loss or grief
- A sense that life is meaningless and has no real purpose

Here is a list of some behavioral indicators of emotional suppression:

- Excessive use of alcohol or drugs, or a sudden urgent need for alcohol or drugs
- Binge eating and overeating
- Not eating or going long periods without food
- Needing to have all the power or give it all away during sex
- Watching endless hours of television or playing video games
- Working nonstop—not being able to relax
- Excessive use of a cell phone, iPad, or computer
- Constantly keeping yourself busy—can't sit still
- Acting as though a painful situation hasn't occurred
- Eating foods or drinks that are stimulating—sugar, salt, or caffeine
- Excessive use of prescription drugs
- Acting overly calm and Zen-like when underneath you are seething with rage
- Withdrawing from social activities
- Loss of interest in sex
- Being a people pleaser
- Always analyzing, thinking, or intellectualizing your experiences
- Denying how you really feel to yourself and others
- Avoidance of activities such as yoga, prayer, therapy, or meditation that require you to go inward

Physical Signs of Suppression

Emotional energy, when not released, has to go somewhere in the body, and so it manifests as physical cues. We can use these physical cues as helpful guides to let us know we are in need of some emotional attention, expression, and healing. Whenever a client shows up at my studio with back pain, I immediately think to myself, "What's going on emotionally for you right now?" And when I ask the right questions, I find that indeed there is something emotional occurring below the surface. The body is a miraculous machine. If you listen and pay attention to your body, it will tell you what it needs and when.

For years I suffered from chronic neck and back pain. At one point I was seeing a physiotherapist at least once a week. Of course, I blamed my neck and back pain on a trillion "outside" things, because I was not aware that my pain was a physical manifestation of my emotional world. Only when I began to *pay attention* and *listen* to my body cues did I discover the emotions that were creating my pain. And it was only when I loved, acknowledged, and released my feelings did my pain simply go away. I still see a chiropractor every now and again, but I have not had chronic neck or back pain since.

I have also witnessed clients heal their physical pain by addressing their emotional needs. One of my clients named Mary used to suffer from chronic urinary tract infections almost every month. After we healed her emotional body, her urinary tract infections only happened every now and again. This is because the mind, body, and spirit are all connected. (We'll talk more about this connection later in the chapter.)

For now, here is a small list of some physical body cues that are really invitations to stop what you are doing, go within, and become aware of what you are feeling:

- Back pain
- Headaches
- General malaise
- Fatigue
- Migraines
- Stiffness

- Stomach pain
- Nausea
- Dizziness
- Muscle aches
- Colds and flu

THOUGHT PROVOKERS

What physical symptoms do you experience regularly?
- *Do you find that certain events or people trigger these symptoms?*
- *Are there any behaviors listed above that resonate with you?*
- *Are you aware of the relationship between your emotional world and your physical body?*
- *Is it easy or challenging for you to relax and do nothing?*
- *What happens for you when you are challenged to face your true feelings?*

The Risks of Emotional Avoidance

Denying and avoiding our emotions for long periods is not only exhausting, it also cages our ability to be free to be who we want to be and is detrimental to our physical, mental, and spiritual health. Suppressing emotions over time requires an enormous amount of effort and energy that zaps vitality, and results in lifeless states such as depression, boredom, and fatigue, as well as illness and an acceleration of the natural aging process.

Laughter and tears are natural bodily functions. Laughter releases happy endorphins and tears serve to detox the body and cleanse it. If you resist your tears, it becomes harder to laugh and feel states of joy and peace. If you are deliberately attempting to be upbeat, without being honest with yourself and others about how you really feel inside, you are repressing a whole range of emotional experiences available to you that are pleasant. Hiding your true emotional self makes it more difficult to access states of unconditional love and motivation—states necessary for taking better care of your health. It also makes is more challenging to have an authentic and unconditionally loving relationship.

When I was depressed in my younger years, I stopped feeling altogether. My soul felt empty and I remember feeling like life had no purpose or meaning. But this was directly due to my emotional suppression. Without our emotions and feelings, how else do we experience our lives? It wasn't until I started to get honest about my true feelings and then lovingly release them that my world, once black and white, became a rainbow of colors again. Suddenly life had purpose and meaning. Life was instantly magnificent!

When we are unhappy, so often we think it's because the circumstances around us need to change. We think we're unhappy because of our weight, our job, our marriage, finances, our divorce, our kids, our inability to have kids, our house, our health, or any number of external circumstances. But if we can allow ourselves to feel the whole range of emotions already inside us, we may find that we are happy already—as well as sad, angry, excited, frightened, and content from time to time. We just weren't allowing ourselves to experience anything but unhappiness. In other words, very often to become happy with your life, you need to make a change on the *inside* rather than the outside.

THOUGHT PROVOKERS

- *Does the world around you change as your feelings change?*
- *Does life sometimes feel void of purpose and meaning?*
- *Do you often look out at the world and wonder what others find so joyful that you can't see?*
- *When you take a quick inventory now of your emotional world, is shame, guilt, fear, or anger present?*

Defining Emotions

Different people define emotions in different ways. For the purpose of this book, I define emotions as powerfully strong energetic forces that are the voice of our souls, which get trapped within our neurology if not released. These energetic impulses that course throughout our bodies are triggered by our experiences—or rather, the thoughts and beliefs we have *about* those experiences. When we have the ability to experience our emotions without judgment and edits, what arises in our experience is the truth of that moment as it's actually being experienced by the soul. When this situation arises, the soul can then learn from the experience and evolve itself to experience something greater—more extraordinary. Emotions are a lot like a GPS. If we pay close attention to the messages inside our emotions, they will guide us in life to what we wish most to experience. But like ignoring the GPS in your car, if you ignore your feelings, you're likely to get lost.

Emotions are what give richness to life. They are not to be feared. They're to be cherished.

Jillian's Story

A few years back, I coached a client named Jillian. Jillian was married and in her forties, and had a teenage son. She was carrying an unhealthy forty additional pounds on her small frame. She was also the CEO of a large medical company, and in addition to a ton of physical symptoms ranging from back pain to migraines, Jillian could never sit still. She constantly felt agitated and anxious— feelings she could avoid as long as she kept herself busy. But she was becoming exhausted and experiencing feelings of apathy and depression.

We went deeply into Jillian's world and we discovered old buried feelings of guilt and shame. When she released those feelings, she became immediately aware of how she'd been living a life she did not want. She had no passion for her medical job and no joy in her life and relationships. But once she let go and released her guilt and shame, she suddenly knew what she wanted. She quit her corporate job to follow her passion in real estate by becoming a real estate agent. She *listened* to the voice of her soul *through* her emotions and began living the life she had always felt in her heart. Naturally, she also lost the weight.

THOUGHT PROVOKERS

- *Are you living the life you'd always dreamed about?*
- *What are you passionate about?*
- *What do you value?*
- *Does your career fulfill you or drain you?*
- *If you had a magic wand and unlimited funds, what would you be doing with your life?*

Acknowledge, Listen to, and Love Your Emotions

Emotions serve a divine and extraordinary purpose. They reveal the truth of our nature, our direct experience of the moment, and what we think and believe about ourselves and circumstances in the moment.

While there is no such thing as a "negative emotion," there are *limiting* emotions, such as anger, guilt, shame, and fear, which serve as a kind of inner alarm system that alerts us to an area within ourselves that needs to be acknowledged, loved unconditionally, and *heard.*

I like to describe our emotional needs similarly to those of a child. When my young son has an emotional experience that leaves him feeling unsafe and afraid, he screams and does whatever he can to get my immediate attention. He is looking to me to reassure him of two primary things: that he is *safe* and he is *loved.* As soon as my little guy *remembers* these things through my attention and loving acknowledgment of his experiences, he stops his loud hollering and goes on his merry way. And because he's a child, the feelings that arise aren't tied to a long history or past, but rather to whatever is arising in the present moment. As he gets older (and it's starting to happen already), he will of course do what we all have done: he will begin to suppress some of his feelings and/or attach other feelings, thoughts, and beliefs to his experiences because of his past. This is part of the "human condition"—until we become *aware.* He will start to experience his present moments based on past moments—*unless* he can learn to let go of his past, be present to what arises emotionally in the moment, and acknowledge, love, and release.

Are you spending any time going "within"?

Ana's Story

Just recently, one of my clients, Ana, an amazing, loving and sensitive gal, shared with me that in the time I've been training and coaching her, she finally reached the realization that she had been living her life from what she described as "the neck up," just as I had many years ago. Like myself, Rosemary (whose story we heard in chapter 1), and so many others I've worked with, she had vacated her body when the emotional pain she felt in her body was too great to bear. Instead of the natural way of life, which is to intuitively *feel* what is right for us at any given moment in time, Ana would spend hours and hours going round and round in her head with the same limiting and discouraging thought patterns.

This constant mental chatter not only drained, confused, and frustrated Ana, but she realized it had prevented her from knowing herself deeply throughout her life. She had never really developed a relationship with *herself*. She didn't know what she liked, what she was passionate about, what her values were, what her opinions on things were, or what it was she really wanted from her life. She knew what everyone else liked and loved but knew nothing about her true self. Of course, as she began to spend more time *in her body*—both physically and in a state of inner reflection and self-inquiry—truths began to emerge from within her that allowed her to start to see *who she really is*.

THOUGHT PROVOKERS

- *Do you spend all your time trapped in your head?*
- *When a problem arises, do you search your head or your heart for the answer?*
- *Do you know what you value and what your opinions on things are?*

- *Do you feel as though you have a voice – that you are able to speak about your feelings?*
- *Do you know with certainty who you really are?*

The emotional energy racing throughout your body is like an internal information highway, carrying messages to and from the body and mind to let you know whether you are in a state of loving homeostasis or not. When you don't pay attention, those emotional messages get louder and more intense. When you eat to suppress them, you further deny their existence, and they cry out in pain and anguish. In response, they push and they push and they do whatever they can to bring your attention back to them. The more you resist, the more they push—and the more you eat and expand (as we'll discuss in more detail below). On the other hand, when you stop, listen, and pay attention to this information, you free yourself to be who you really are. When you tend to your emotions in a space of loving awareness, your body, mind, and soul can return to its natural state of peace and contentment. And you no longer feel the impulse to eat.

Your Emotions Are a Direct Pathway Back to the Soul

As such, our emotions serve as a direct pathway back to the soul, the eternal part of ourselves that's in direct communication with the Infinite Wisdom and our own awareness of how to best live our lives fearlessly and joyfully. The soul knows that we are intimately connected not only to one another, but also to the divine greatness that loves, guides, and supports us all. This Infinite Wisdom and awareness goes by many names: some call it Source, Spirit, Oneness, the Universe, the Creator, or God.

Unfortunately the word "God" these days triggers a lot of negative feelings for many people, especially if they were raised in a strict religious environment where "God" was something to be feared, and would punish, humiliate, or stop loving you for a multitude of reasons—none of which is true, by the way. If this understanding of God resonates with you, the word "God" should be tossed from your vocabulary. Whatever name you want to give to the Infinite Wisdom—the love and beauty of life—does not matter at all. Nor does the Infinite Wisdom care, as we humans might, what name you wish to call it. All that matters to the Infinite Wisdom is that you know you are loved and that you matter, and that life becomes easier and more joyful when you let this Infinite Wisdom guide your life *through* your heart and emotions.

Personally, I like the word God—but then I wasn't raised in an environment where God was menacing. For me, the word God is synonymous with unconditional love, and so when I think about God, I feel immense love, not fear. However, I have clients and family members who had different and limiting religious experiences, so the word "God" sends them running for the hills. This is so heartbreaking and unfortunate, as it can cause us to shut down our divine relationship to the Infinite Wisdom within ourselves and miss out on the loving guidance and support it wants to bring to our lives. I personally could not have conquered all the inner demons, challenges, and struggles I have experienced without the love and support of God. I accomplish all that I do *because* of my relationship with God.

THOUGHT PROVOKERS

- *Does the discussion of God trigger any thoughts and feelings within you?*
- *What thoughts and feelings are triggered?*
- *Do you believe in a Higher Power, but you're not yet certain of how this Higher Power affects you?*
- *Has there been a time in your life when you felt the immense loving presence of something more than yourself?*
- *Do you know you are loved beyond measure just as you are, or does this truth make you feel uncomfortable?*
- *Do you believe you are safe and being taken care of?*

We talked earlier in this book about the mental roadblocks that create resistance to thinking about and perceiving our experiences in new ways.

Similarly, emotional roadblocks create a detour away from the positive lessons emotional states can offer us. Emotional roadblocks also prevent us from experiencing the richness available through expressing emotions. But we need to identify and conquer these emotional roadblocks so we can feel and express our truth—or we'll forever be trapped inside a body that suppresses us.

Eating Your Feelings

As I said at the very beginning of the chapter, one major reason you are challenged with your weight is due to your relationship with food—you are using food as therapy instead of fuel. Yes, it's true that diet and exercise are also factors in weight management, but if you are using food as a means to cope emotionally, the importance of diet and exercise combined pales in comparison. The biggest problem is that your *emotions*, not true hunger, motivate you to eat. Your emotions trigger your craving for sugary, salty foods that you know intellectually are bad for you.

In fact, emotional stress can cause your weight to fluctuate like crazy, even if you have not made any changes to your food and exercise regimen. Many times I have witnessed clients gain weight one week and then lose it all the next when the only thing that changed was how they were managing their emotional stress. When emotions are held in, they gained weight. When released, they lost weight. Even the mere act of constantly *thinking* about food can create unnecessary feelings of stress and anxiety when clients believe that without food they will not be safe.

As I mentioned earlier, there is no such thing as a "negative" or "positive" emotion. All emotions serve a positive purpose, although there are some emotions that limit our life experiences *only* if held onto for too long and not released. Depression, anger, rage, resentment, envy, shame, guilt, and hurt are all examples of emotions that, when buried deep inside for too long, result in a joyless and passionless life. Even these emotional experiences, when we let them, provide a divine opportunity for us to learn, evolve, and grow, and ultimately to become the person we want to be.

In the Mood for Food

Food cravings are triggered by mood more than hunger. A need for love and attention can feel like a need for food. But when we stop turning to food for love, we turn to ourselves instead, and the feeling of love from ourselves far outweighs the feeling of love we get from food.

Start recognizing cravings as signals that indicate you have a deeper need that is not getting met—LOVE.

The reasons we eat are emotional 90 percent of the time. Studies now reveal that certain emotional states can even be linked to eating certain foods. For example, we tend to gravitate toward crunchy foods like potato chips when we feel angry and softer foods like ice cream when we feel sad or alone.[13] Whenever I get sad and need a little loving, I instantly want to inhale a box of chocolate, or even better, throw down a hot and creamy Thai curry. Just thinking about the curry and the chocolate ignites the belief in me that the food will make me feel better—except it doesn't. In every moment of every day we are *always* looking for what will make us feel better. What will improve this moment? What will change how I feel? Too often, the answer is . . . "Food!" Even if it's a box of old stale potato chips we find in the bottom of the pantry, it does the job of suppressing our true feelings. I can remember a time when I was feeling empty of love and I ate a three-day-old pizza that hadn't even been refrigerated! It had been sitting on my counter gathering dust—and Lord only knows what else— but I inhaled it as if my life depended on it!

We Don't Take Pills—We Eat!

Food has become a socially acceptable and common form of self-medication. Just as the pharmaceutical industry tells us that popping a pill will take care of our depressing and anxious feelings, we like to tell ourselves that eating will also numb our depression and anxiety and suppress the emotions we don't want to feel – like boredom. All it really does is suppress our *symptoms* without ever addressing the cause—just like pharmaceutical drugs! We knock ourselves out with a massive carb load that makes us feel like we're drunk, so we no longer have to think, and that food acts like a drug that quells the pain. At some point, we develop an addiction that we purposely participate in to avoid having to deal with the real reason for why we feel so emotionally shitty!

THOUGHT PROVOKERS

- *What emotional experiences drive you to eat?*
- *What foods do you gravitate toward when emotional?*
- *Do you find you eat different foods based on how you're feeling?*
- *Does emotional stress cause you to gain weight (or lose it) without changing your diet?*
- *If you're on a pharmaceutical, has it resolved your unhappiness, or are you just simply able to function?*
- *Can you recall a funny story when you ate something like a three-day-old pizza?*
- *Can you laugh at yourself as you recall this memory and love yourself for being human?*
- *Are you becoming more aware now of how you use food to soothe?*

Nadine's Story

When Nadine first came to see me, she was trapped inside forty pounds of unnecessary fat. She was depressed to her core, wanted to kill herself, and had been on antidepressant and anti-anxiety medication for years. In less than a year of doing the "inner work" of facing and releasing old emotional wounds, she found she no longer needed her meds and gradually weaned herself off them. She not only stopped using food to cope, she also stopped using pharmaceutical medications. She discovered her truth and now lives it.

Studies and Research Confirm Emotions Impact Health

Studies and research now confirm what many of us have intuitively understood for years—in addition to having a more limited experience of life, people who repress, ignore, or deny their emotions are often wide-open targets for physical illness. Every emotion has a particular energetic vibration, and the emotions we typically call "negative," such as anger, fear, anxiety, frustration, or depression, have a lower vibration than "positive" emotions, such as joy, love, acceptance, compassion, and forgiveness. Over time, lower-vibrating emotions that don't get expressed and released, but stay buried within our energetic and physical bodies, create chemical reactions in the body that in turn can cause serious physical breakdowns and disease, including cancers, heart problems, obesity, diabetes, hormonal imbalances, chronic fatigue, and chronic pain conditions like fibromyalgia. In contrast, storing higher-vibrating, positive emotions in our bodies creates a very different chemical reaction that in turn generates health, wellness, and well-being.

Studies are also revealing now that certain types of suppressed emotions can be correlated to certain physical dysfunctions. For example, liver problems can be connected to suppressed rage and anger—information, by the way, that Chinese medicine has understood and taught for thousands of years. Louise Hay, the pioneer of positive thinking and founder of Hay House Publishing, whose influence I grew up under as a child, has been saying this same thing for decades. For instance, in her book *Heal Your Body*, she lists a number of physical ailments, their corresponding thought patterns, and a suggested new thought pattern that is more empowering and healing. Under the category of "overweight," Hay suggests the probable causes are: "fear, need for protection, and running away from feelings, as well as insecurity, self-rejection, and seeking fulfillment." She suggests the following new thought patterns as a means to evoke new emotional experiences and freedom: "I am at peace with my own feelings. I am safe where I am. I create my own security. I love and approve of myself."[14]

Emotional Sensitivity

I have heard and read that people who are overweight are "emotionally sensitive." But in truth, we are *all* emotionally sensitive, which isn't a problem but a blessing. Our emotional sensitivity only becomes a problem when we suppress it, whether through food, drugs, sex, alcohol, "busyness," or any number of ways.

I myself am emotionally sensitive. But whereas this sensitivity used to be unbearable at times, this same sensitivity now affords me the ability to *empower and heal others.* It sometimes still overwhelms me, but it also allows me to experience a richer, more expansive, and divine experience of life. Emotional sensitivity should *not* be viewed as a disorder or a weakness. It should be viewed as a gift.

THOUGHT PROVOKERS

- *How do you feel about your thoughts and feelings affecting your physical body?*
- *Does this make you feel powerful or powerless?*
- *Do you resonate with being "emotionally sensitive?"*

Everything's Okay—You're Okay

As children, it's very likely that any time you experienced discomfort, pain, or fear, you were given food, probably something sugary like cookies and ice cream, and those treats made you feel happier and comforted. Then at some point you made a mental and physiological connection between feeling pain, fear, or discomfort, and the realization that if you eat, you can feel better. Now, every time you feel emotionally out of control or overwhelmed, you know from past experience that if you eat something sugary, salty, or loaded with carbs, at least in that moment of eating, it will bring some feelings of comfort and relief. When those feelings are soothed, we feel momentarily stronger and better able to deal with whatever's happening in the present. In other words, even though you don't want to eat and you know it's going to make you feel worse afterwards, it's easier to mask the feelings of disappointment, guilt, failure, etc. with food than it is to deal with the root-cause emotions you are suppressing. However, it is far more empowering and healing to learn how to cope with our emotions more effectively, in a process of love, awareness, grace, learning, and acceptance, rather than masking them with food.

You may think, "But I know all this—why can't I stop this behavior?"

The key is in the previous sentence: "a process of love, awareness, grace, learning, and acceptance." You can only effectively cope with your emotions in a context of love and acceptance. I want you to see that, even up to this moment, you have taken care of yourself remarkably well. You may be forty or sixty or one hundred pounds (or more) overweight, but hear me when I say that you did the best you could with the resources you had and currently have available to you. You could only operate from within the programming you downloaded as a child and the awareness you currently have. Once you courageously look within yourself, and lovingly release the old, suppressed emotions and patterns of avoidance you developed as survival strategies, only then will you be able to stop the behavior of unhealthy eating. The strategies that once felt like they protected you and served you are no longer needed and are now blocking your growth. It is time to let go and move on.

At this point in our lives, food is the substitute for the love and peace we lost inside, the love we believe we should have received, in most cases, from our parents or those we love most in our lives. When we feel this lack of love, we feel afraid, and when we feel afraid, we feel like we're going to die. I know this sounds dramatic, but it's true! (We'll talk more about fear and how the fight or flight response works in chapter 8.) We will do anything to survive, and we will gravitate to whatever it is we learned early on in our life that reduces or alleviates the feeling of fear. We use food as our comfort and coping mechanism, and as a way to control and suppress our fears.

The greatest lie we tell ourselves is that we do not have the inner resources, courage, or resilience to survive our emotional pain. But I assure you that you do. I survived. My clients survived. You will survive too. And not only will you survive your emotions, but they will also free you and strengthen you in ways you can't imagine.

Emotional Addiction

As I mentioned at the beginning of the chapter, it is important to identify the root-cause emotions that are truly fueling our unhealthy relationship with food. However, not all of the negative emotions we feel are root-cause emotions. Many of us can more easily recognize what I like to refer to as "coping" emotions, or the secondary or tertiary emotions that are symptoms of the root-cause emotions. These include emotional states such as anger, frustration, depression, stoicism, confusion, guilt, and boredom—feelings we'd prefer to feel instead of what is really going on for us emotionally.

When we find ourselves regularly engaging in these coping emotions, it is often because we have become *addicted* to the chemical responses they produce in the body. Expressing these symptomatic emotions becomes a substitute for expressing our deepest, true emotions. Many people will engage in anger, for instance, as a means to avoid vulnerability and expressing their hurt. For those of us who use food as a coping mechanism for our coping emotions, the more we engage in these coping emotions, the more we literally "feed" our addiction. This is very similar to what happens with an addiction to alcohol: those who drink too much as a means to cope emotionally are not only addicted to the coping emotion, but to the chemical responses from the alcohol itself, continuing to drink only fuels both addictions. You usually have to stop drinking altogether to end the cycle. But we can't stop eating food, obviously, so instead we have to find other ways to produce the same, if not better, chemical responses we get from the food we have become addicted to. We'll talk more about how to do this in Part 2, where we discuss your optimal nutrition plan. But the first step is to break the underlying addiction to your coping emotions, cease suppressing our emotions, and allow those root-cause emotions to surface.

When we don't allow our emotions to surface and release as they are naturally designed to do, it creates unnecessary suffering, as I know you are now fully aware. I know it can feel scary to express your truth and be vulnerable, but it's the only way you're going to transform.

Letting Go

Remember, our emotions are gifts to be treasured and felt, not buried and hidden out of sight. Our emotions are a huge part of who we are, and they are meant to ebb and flow, arise, disappear, come and go, peak and dissolve. When you say *no* to your emotions, you don't just bury *them*, you also bury *you*—your beautiful truth and divine uniqueness, which will benefit the world if you allow it. My reader, you are extraordinary! You matter and you're here for a purpose—to be exactly *who you are!* If you don't let go and heal your emotions, then you are ignoring the deepest most authentic, spiritual part of who you are.

The Truth Will Set You Free

The good news is our emotions cannot remain buried inside us forever, because truth always surfaces eventually. Yes, this *is* good news, even if it may not seem so right now. You can help this process go more smoothly, or you can attempt to walk the path I took (and I do not recommend it, by the way), which was to kick, scream, fight, and resist my truth. You should know that I'm a pretty tough cookie. So if I failed miserably (and gratefully, as it's turned out), then it's likely you are going to fail trying to resist too—which is a good thing, since you *want* the truth of who you are to come out.

Your "truth" is wrapped up inside your true emotions, and these emotions will do whatever they can to find their way to get your attention. You can try to run from your emotions by continuing to eat everything in sight, move to a new house or even to a new country, and ditch one relationship for another in the hope of a new experience. You can smoke, you can have sex, you can masturbate until your hand falls off or watch hours of pornography, you can get drunk, high, or stare for hours at your iPad, but nothing—I repeat, *nothing*—will stop your suppressed emotions from eventually arising. So you may as well put down the gloves, and stop fighting a battle that holds only empty promises and is one you cannot ever win.

Love Is the Best Food Ever!

Love really *is* the answer. I know it sounds cheesy, and might even make you queasy, but it is what it is, so accept it. The beauty of your emotional body blossoms as you love yourself unconditionally and allow yourself be loved unconditionally by God, the Universe, and the people who love you. As you allow yourself to give and receive more love, you will discover just how often you ignore your emotions to "push through" and move on. You will see how often you neglect, abuse, and abandon yourself, and while it will likely be heart wrenching at first to acknowledge, the acknowledgment will change the way you treat yourself. When I first came to this awareness myself, I bawled for hours, saying only the words, "I am sorry. I love you. I forgive you. I am sorry."

Elizabeth's Story

When I met Elizabeth, she was forty-three years old and about ninety pounds overweight. She had moved from California to Canada with three children and was extremely unhappy. Her marriage was stressed to the limit and she desperately missed her friends and family back in California. The way Elizabeth described her emotional state was, "I feel like I'm always about to lose it at any second, but with three children to take care of I can't afford to do that. I don't have the time." So instead, she stuffed her emotions down (what many mamas do, I might add), pretended they didn't exist, and ate excessively unhealthy foods to cope.

Elizabeth's feelings of loss and sadness were so overwhelming that she often felt compelled to go to the grocery store several times a day and even during the night to get candy bars and potato crisps just to keep herself sane. She admitted that while she felt lousy about eating the way she did, it at least stopped her from feeling like she was going to fall apart.

More than anything, Elizabeth did not want to fall apart. She was afraid that if she busted a gut expressing all her frustrations and fears and grief, all emotional hell would break loose. She was trying so hard to keep it all together that her only outlet was rushing to the store and filling her face with candy bars. Sound familiar to anyone? Does it make anything better? Of course not.

It wasn't until Elizabeth gave herself permission during our sessions to release what she had suppressed for so long that she was finally able to move forward with her life. With more love and appreciation for herself, she began taking better care of her health. Having released her emotional burdens, Elizabeth suddenly had more energy, vitality, confidence, lightness, and self-esteem. Now she lives in greater awareness of what her emotional and physical body actually need. When old cravings come up, she knows something inside her needs her care and attentiveness. She listens, she loves, and she does her best to provide what she needs for herself.

THOUGHT PROVOKERS

- *What do you think when you hear the words, "love yourself"?*
- *Are there some parts of you that you love, and others that you don't?*
- *If you allow yourself, even for just a tiny second, to be loved unconditionally, how does it feel?*
- *Do you dish your love out to others—but when it comes to yourself, think, "Oh, that's different"?*
- *Do you think God (Source, Spirit, Jesus, the Universe, your Higher Power) loves you unconditionally?*

Don't Be Afraid to Feel

I finally let out all my feelings in my mid-twenties. As I often tell my clients, it felt like I bawled my eyes out for two years straight, which is a slight exaggeration, but not too far from the truth. Through my tears I expressed anger, hurt, resentments, guilt, fear, shame—you name it! Once I released it all, however, I felt like an entirely different person. I felt free. Even now I continue to feel lighter and happier as I allow my emotions to come forward and release from moment to moment. They evaporate like raindrops and I return to my higher awareness. I see that they are relevant in the moment but not worth keeping around. I would rather acknowledge them now than accumulate a jumble of confused emotions and try to deal with them later.

However, I had to hit rock bottom before I was desperate enough to willingly let go of what felt like a thousand years' worth of emotional baggage. This is not a pathway I wish on anyone, by the way, but it does appear to be the most common. It is human nature to wait until the pain of suppressing becomes greater than the pain of expressing. And that's okay. When we are ready to let go, we will—each in our own good time. But you don't have to go to the depths of despair, as I did. Start from where you are now. And if you are already in the depths of despair, then I'm here to tell you that you can start here too.

Awareness (Again)

The first step to releasing suppressed emotions is simply to bring awareness, attention, and love to whatever you feel in the moment. Often, this attention alone will change what we feel. Rather than doing what I originally suggested in my book, *Manage Your Mind, Master Your Life*, and what other well-meaning, self-help books suggest you do, which is to change what you feel to something more "positive" or "better," I invite you instead to simply welcome and acknowledge your feelings. Just allow whatever wants to be expressed, to be expressed. Bring some love and acceptance to whatever you feel. Let it be okay and know it won't last forever. Then once you have acknowledged your presenting emotions, now you can access and manifest new and more empowering emotional states like certainty, motivation, joy, or love, simply by choosing and intending it and by reframing your thoughts and focus in that moment. And when you can let be what will be, what happens next feels like a miracle. You'll transform.

Here are some practices to engage in, so you can begin becoming more aware of your emotional world and heal what needs to healed within you.

Practices: The Heart of the Matter

Going Deeper

Often when we haven't yet learned how to welcome and then release our emotions, the emotion that first surfaces is a secondary, sometimes tertiary, emotional symptom of the real emotion that needs to be unearthed and addressed. So the next time you become aware of an emotion, stop what you're doing if able, close your eyes, and go within. Identify the emotion you're experiencing and then imagine that you can gently fall through this emotion to an even deeper emotion that lies beneath. At each emotional level, welcome the emotion that reveals itself to you, ask what it wants you to know, then thank it, release it, and drop down another layer.

In many instances when you do this, you'll discover that you eventually find yourself feeling an emotion of calm, peace, love, and oneness. If, however, you find yourself hitting an emotional wall you can't fall though, and you're not experiencing an emotion of calm, peace, love, or oneness, this is a beautiful indication that some healing of this particular emotion is required. Journal this observation and meditate on it until the information you need to know, in order to release, arises in your conscious awareness. If this doesn't happen and you still can't release, consider seeking the guidance of a professional therapist or practitioner who can assist you with the process. Sometimes we need the involvement of another person or persons to help us breathe through our blind spots and find clarity.

Journaling

On a daily basis, preferably when you retire to bed at night, write down how you felt during the day. Were there times you felt discouraged and angry, and other times you felt peaceful and calm. Whatever your emotional experiences were that day, make detailed notes in your journal. Then reflect on these emotions and self-inquire as to what deeper emotions may lie beneath. You can use the above and below practices to help you move through the emotions you experience.

Emotional Release Practice

If a disconcerting emotion arises within you, instead of trying to resist and avoid it, say "hello" to your feelings and acknowledge their existence. Ask them what messages they have for you and what they want you to know. Ask them what they need to feel (e.g., safety, love, acceptance, or understanding) in order for you to allow them to be released. Then repeat the statement below, which is an adaptation of the Emotional Freedom Technique (EFT) developed by Gary Craig in the early 1990s, while simultaneously tapping the points between your eyebrows with your first and second fingers until the intensity of the emotion either reduces and/or vanishes.

Even though I feel (insert whatever you are feeling), I know I am safe and loved unconditionally by God (or Source or Spirit or whichever name resonates with you), and I deeply and completely love and accept myself. All is well. I am at peace.

Emotional Body Scanning

At least once a day, spend time being fully present to your body. Go into a relaxing meditation and mentally scan your entire body from your toes to your head, noticing any emotional energies being stored there. When you notice an emotion, send it love and acceptance. Invite it to share with you what it wants you to know. Then say thank you to the emotion, and ask it to leave your body.

Emotional Eating Awareness Exercise

The next time you find yourself reaching for a tub of ice cream or unable to stop yourself from eating the entire pizza, consider these two questions, and then journal your observations and tell at least one other person:

If what I am about to eat were an emotion and not a food, what emotion would I be eating?

and

What am I feeling right now that I don't want to feel, and that I've come to learn through experience will go away at least temporarily, if I just eat this tub of ice cream or the rest of this pizza?

Loving What Is

This practice is my favorite practice and, when practiced regularly, has great power to positively transform your life in a radical and divinely enriching way.

Whenever you observe any emotion arise, instead of judging it, critiquing it, editing it, labeling it, trying to figure it out, or understand it, just love it, thank it, and then release it. Sometimes emotions and feelings will arise and you'll immediately know what they are about and what their message for you is, especially if you practice the above—and this is wonderful. But sometimes emotions and feelings just surface, and we have no conscious awareness of their origin, purpose, or intent. In these instances, it is especially effective to simply love what is, through the power of attention, presence, unconditional love, and acceptance, and then release. My understanding about these unknown feelings is that we are not necessarily meant to "get into the detail." It is simply our mental, emotional, and physical body cleansing itself of what it no longer needs to experience. We don't need to understand it, nor do we need to have all the information in order to experience the healing benefits. All that's required is to simply let go.

Find a "Share Your Feelings" Buddy

I have an amazing girlfriend named Donna who lives in Australia, whom I've known for many years now and who has journeyed along this life with me, privy to all that I have gone through and experienced. There hasn't been much we have not told each other about what's going on in our lives—much like many girlfriends' experiences. But recently, in this last year, Donna and I decided to take our relationship once step further. We agreed to be totally and utterly transparent with one another and to share our deepest and truest feelings with each other, under the agreement that we would simply love the other person and their experience without any judgment. Imagine if there was someone in your life with whom you were able to share the inner most parts of your soul. I assure you, it is liberating, enlightening, and deeply enriching.

I invite you to find your "Donna." Choose a person whom you love deeply, trust implicitly, and ask them to be your "Donna." At least once a month (if you don't live in the same location), connect with your Donna and release. Get everything out. Lay your emotional cards on the table. Show up in your naked truth and set yourself free. If you feel you do not have a Donna, I highly recommend a heart-centered therapist or coach who will provide a loving space for you to speak your truth and be free.

CHAPTER 6

SELF-LOVE: A BEAUTIFUL TRUTH

You can search throughout the entire universe for someone who is more deserving of your love and affection than you are yourself, and that person is not to be found anywhere. You yourself, as much as anybody in the entire universe, deserve your love and affection.
Buddha

Taken together, both this chapter and the previous one form the true heart of the matter when it comes to weight loss and becoming who you are destined to be. Once you begin to express rather than suppress your emotions, as you discovered how to do in the previous chapter, you become able to develop the quality that will start to fuel true, lasting success in transforming your body and your life from the inside out. This quality is *self-love*. Only when you are able to love yourself *as you are* will you be naturally able to do all that is required to care for your body in the ways it needs to thrive. But as simple as it sounds, most people find this to be the most difficult step of all.

Here's how I know. When I meet with clients for the first time, I invite them to stand in front of a full-length mirror and share with me what they see. I do this because I'm interested in what their health and fitness expectations are, but more importantly, I do it because I am interested in seeing how much (or how little) they respect and care about themselves. As their trainer and coach, I hold a loving space for my clients to learn to love *themselves*. It's easy to do. I hold my love for them in my heart and I visualize this love leaving my body and entering into theirs. When I enter my studio, I fill it with my love. I want every person who walks through my studio doors to know they are welcome and loved.

What clients share through their words and body language, as they look in the mirror, allows me some insight into their view of themselves as well as their *love language*—the way in which they love or don't love themselves on a regular basis. Their answers reveal their perceptions of themselves, their view of the world around them, as well as their expectations and judgments. It's important for me to know this because *how we communicate to ourselves* plays a significant role in our body's ability to heal, lose weight and transform.

The messages you give to your body shape your body.

True health and wellness is a combination of mental, emotional, spiritual, and physical well-being. To achieve this total well-being, we need love. I know everyone wants a fit and fabulous body they can feel proud of—I do, too! But it's important that we also understand that our *physical* appearance is not a measure of our worth or a prerequisite for receiving unconditional love—rather, it is a by-product.

True health and wellness is about *balance*—the balance of love, health, and harmony across our mental, emotional, spiritual, and physical selves. To achieve this, we need to have a loving flame that burns brightly and continuously within us. Believe me, I know a lot of men and women with very fit and fabulous looking physiques who are far from what I'd consider *healthy* and who have become addicted to their outer appearance to the point of obsession. Their outer appearance may look fantastic, but inside they're a mess mentally, emotionally, and spiritually.

True beauty stems from the inside out.

The goal of true wellness is to create beauty and health on the *inside* first. And what is beauty, really, but *love?* Love is what attracts people to each other, and love is really what everyone wants! Your body doesn't *need* to look like the fitness models on the front of magazines. Hours and hours of preparation, make-up, and lighting has gone into those images to make them appear flawless, which is really quite ridiculous when you think about it, since *nobody* on the planet can have a body that looks like that in real life. So all that you should be focusing on is creating the best body you can with the amazing body you've got!

No two bodies are alike, nor were they intended to be.

It's also important to remind yourself that bodies come in all shapes and sizes. If you have broad shoulders and wide hips, it's futile to stand in front of a mirror and wish for a different body shape. You can pray for months on a mountaintop, but nothing's going to change the physical structure of your body. Nor should you want it to, as it's your body for a reason. Plus this type of unrealistic expectation will only frustrate and upset you. It's sending damaging messages to your body that say, "Hey, you're not good enough," which is completely disempowering and soul-destroying, not to mention demotivating. When was the last time you felt motivated and excited to work out and eat right after being told who you are is not good enough?

Your body is a beautiful gift. Treat it with love and it will love you back.

Your body is perfect, and it's time for you to begin realizing so. If you have broad hips and shoulders, learn to love your broad hips and shoulders. If you're like me and you have hardly any hips at all, then learn to love your hips just as they are. If you've got long legs, love them! If you're got short legs, love them, too! If you have big breasts, love 'em! If you have small breasts, love them with all your heart! Learning to love your body shape just as it is sends messages to your body of love, gratitude, and acceptance—all the states we need to motivate ourselves to take excellent care of ourselves.

To dream of the body you'd like to have is to waste the body you already have.

Arlene's Story

I once trained a client named Arlene. Arlene was an artist—tall, beautiful, and in her late twenties. Arlene would drive me crazy because at the start of every training session, she'd ask me what I could do to *shrink* the size of her hips. Time and time again I'd tell her, "Arlene, your hips are your natural body shape and no amount of exercise is going to change your structural shape. Secondly, and for the trillionth time this month, you must stop compartmentalizing and judging your body shape, because your body is beautiful, for crying out loud, and your narrow view of yourself is preventing you from seeing your magnificence!" Of course, the response I often get back is, "But isn't this why I am here—to *change* my body?" "No!" I reply. "It's not why you're here. You're here to love your body and yourself *as you are,* and from there we focus on transforming your body into the best body it can be. And this does not mean a surgical reduction of your hips, which I remind you again are BEAUTIFUL!"

Change your view of yourself, not your shape.

Of course I have many "Arlenes" who train with me (sometimes I myself fall into the trap of being an "Arlene"), and I remind them all, as I remind myself, that we were given the bodies we have because they are perfect for who we are destined to be in this life, and once we stop criticizing, abusing, and hurting our bodies, only then will we be able to transform them into the best bodies they can be. To transform our bodies, we must *love* our bodies and realize our bodies aren't a curse, but a gift.

When my clients first stand in front of the full-length mirror and tell me what they see, some of their responses are heartbreaking and are exactly what drive them to abandon their bodies, eat to excess or starve themselves nearly to death. These responses are also the reasons why they struggle to transform their bodies. Hate messages don't motivate—they cause you to stagnate.

Below are some actual statements that clients have shared. See if any of these statements are ones you have said to yourself and recall how they made you *feel*. Imagine saying these same things to your best girlfriend, your parents, or your children! I know you never would, because they're so hurtful and damaging!

- "I cannot believe this is me. Yuck"
- "Ugh. This exercise is making me angry. How is this supposed to help me?"
- "I don't want to look at myself in the mirror! I don't want to look at myself!"
- "I see rolls and rolls of fat on my stomach and fat, cellulite-infused legs that rub together."
- "I see flabby arms that look disgusting. And I hate this fat around my ankles. Oh God, I look so old . . . "
- "I hate this stupid exercise! I don't want to look at myself."
- "What does this have to do with losing weight?"

- "I hate you right now . . .this exercise sucks!"
- "I need a coffee. . ."
- "I see a fat face, bad skin, no chin, a sagging bottom—um, what else. . .?"
- "Nothing. I see nothing at all. What am I supposed to be seeing?"
- "Gross! All I see is grossness. I feel sick. I need to use the bathroom."
- "I see someone who should be taking better of herself but doesn't."
- "Ooh, yuck! I'd rather look at you in the mirror!"
- "I see someone who is a bit overweight, but not too bad." (This client was obese.)
- "I see fat everywhere. I need to lose weight here, here, here, and here." (This client was skin and bones.)
- Some people don't speak at all—they just cover their eyes and cry.

We'll have the chance to do several more exercises at the end of the chapter, but I'd like you to try this one right now. Stand in front of a mirror in your home and write down in your journal what *you* see. Start to shed some light on the ways in which you repeatedly talk to yourself. Are you sending yourself love messages or messages that are hateful, judgmental, critical and disempowering? Are you throwing away your power by choosing to berate your body and not to love yourself unconditionally?

Now look at the list of statements about yourself you wrote in your journal, and repeat the following. (Please don't think intellectually about this portion of the exercise, just do it and notice what happens.)

Read your first statement aloud. Pause, then say to yourself,

I am sorry. I love you. I forgive you.

Repeat for each statement.

What Is Self-Love, Really?

When I first began my healing journey, I went to counseling and was invited by my therapist at the time to stand in front of mirror daily and say the words

"I love you." I almost threw up on his sofa. The idea of *loving myself* made me feel so uncomfortable, I wanted to reach across the room and slap him for suggesting such a ridiculous idea. Loving myself? What an absurd thing to do! What did that even mean? And what did loving myself have to do with all the problems I was facing? Naturally, I told myself my therapist was a lunatic and I was best served looking for another one who was going to focus on *fixing* my problems like a good therapist should, not having me stand in front of a mirror saying, "Michelle, I love you." Instantly I felt like I needed a cigarette. However I soon came to realize that when I started loving myself, it became easy to accept the love from those around me and the love that had always been available to me from the Universe (God).

If loving yourself makes you want to vomit, then you're exactly where you're meant to be.

When many people think about loving themselves, it can evoke feelings of discomfort and uneasiness. But that's because we often think of loving ourselves as arrogant or selfish, or just downright stupid and embarrassing. But self-love isn't about stroking the ego or waving a flag that says, *Hey look at me, I'm so awesome!* It's about learning how to take care of yourself in loving ways, taking responsibility for your life, and expressing the truth inside you that makes you who you are.

Many of us have been brought up with the idea that it's okay to love other people unconditionally—our friends, our parents, our children, even our pets. We accept that it's okay to pour our love into our pets and the people around us we love, speaking to them kindly and taking care of them in loving and nurturing ways, yet when it comes to ourselves, we somehow don't deserve the same treatment. This is a huge misconception, since we *all* deserve unconditional love for no other reason than just being ourselves.

Luckily for me, I wasn't able to find another therapist who was willing to agree with my notions on love, and I soon realized, thank goodness, that none of my problems would ever go away if I didn't learn to love myself first.

Love changes everything.

Marianne's Story

When Marianne and I first met approximately one year ago, she was seventy pounds heavier than she is today. She was tired of different diet programs and exercise regimens whose results lasted only temporarily. She was tired of fighting a never-ending battle. She just wanted to be free to live a good life. So not only did Marianne transform her physical self, she also transformed her heart—*literally.*

Before Marianne began training with me, she had many health issues, one being the enlargement of four of her beautiful heart chambers. This obviously concerned Marianne, as it also did me. It put her at risk for imminent heart problems and possibly a shortened life. But after a year of nutrition counseling and workouts with me, in addition to Marianne taking the time to *go within* to do her "inner workouts" (which were equally as important), her cardiologist revealed that three of her heart chambers had returned to normal size and the fourth was well on its way. Yet while Marianne's physical heart was shrinking to a normal size, her spiritual heart and love for herself was expanding!

Here is how Marianne described the process of allowing love back into her heart.

"Since training with Michelle, I have become aware of how I communicate with myself and I have learned to listen to my body and my feelings. I do not want to hide in my body anymore, and with Michelle's guidance and support, I began looking at the root of my struggle with my weight. I asked myself, 'Why do I give in to food? Why do I frequently choose food over my

well-being? What am I so afraid of?' And with great trepidation, I allowed myself to be vulnerable and opened up my heart. By doing so, I felt free to heal and grow.

I do not always understand how I feel or why I do what I do, but I am learning to be kinder and more loving to myself. I am now my best friend, and I am learning to treat myself the same way I would treat someone I love or care about. I have become much better at not letting others' feelings and behaviors get to me. Michelle always reminded me to assure myself: 'Other people's downfalls are not of my concern.' I am not perfect, nor are others. We are all doing the best we can. I've also learned that within me there is a young child who needs my love often, and I give it to her now, when I once did not. Not with food, though. She is much happier with the unconditional love and acceptance I offer."

When you let love in to every fiber of your being, the emotional pain inside of you will heal. Then, as time goes on and more love fills you, the need to eat for love and comfort will subside as an issue in your life. What used to seem difficult—such as exercising regularly and eating healthy meals—suddenly seems easier now and is enjoyable for you, and not a chore. When love fills your heart again, you'll have appreciation for what you see staring back at you from the mirror. Instead of scanning your body for its flaws, you will see your body as a beautiful whole. If you don't let love in, it will destroy you and distort your true view of yourself.

The best food in the world is love.

Without Love

Body Dysmorphia, more commonly known as Body Dysmorphic Disorder (BDD), is medically considered to be a type of mental illness where the "affected" person is overly concerned with their body image, has manifested excessive concern about their body image, and who has an ongoing preoccupation with perceived defects of their physical features that results in significant psychological distress that impairs social functioning, self-esteem, and confidence. Often people dealing with BDD also experience anxiety, depression, social withdrawal, and unhealthy eating habits and treatment of their bodies. The onset of BDD usually occurs in adolescence or early adulthood. It begins with self-criticism of their personal appearance and builds over time until the person is unable to see anything other than their perceived flaws and defects. BDD is prolonged due to ongoing self-abuse.

Self-love, my liege, is not so vile a sin as self-neglecting.
William Shakespeare

Anyone who looks in the mirror and is unable to see past their physical self to their true magnificence has, in my opinion, some form of BDD. This includes people who have fit bodies and physiques as well. But because I think diagnoses like this tend to perpetuate the limiting belief that "there is something wrong with me," when I am working with clients, I refer to this perception of self as the ASLE—the Absence of Self Love Experience. The clients whose comments I shared from the mirror exercise have, in my opinion, ASLE. They are not accurately seeing the truth of themselves. They can't see the totality of who they are. They cannot see their beautiful souls. They only see the physical.

My imperfections and failures are as much a blessing from God as my successes and my talents, and I lay them both at his feet.
Ghandi

Your Flaws Are Beautiful

For me, the most attractive part of a person is their scars. Physical scars from accidents in childhood or later in life are my favorite aspects of a person's body. I'm also attracted to wrinkles. The reason I love scars and wrinkles is because they tell a story about a person's life and because they speak the naked truth of who they really are. I am deeply attracted to authenticity, transparency, and truth (I think we all are when we think about it deeply enough), and when a person's body reflects their truth, to me it's both divine and beautiful. On my own body I have a scar from an emergency C-section I had to have to bring my baby boy into this world. I love this scar, as it always reminds me of the moment my son entered my life. What a blessing!

To Be Human *Is* to Be Flawed

At some point along our human journey we collectively decided it made good sense to try to remove any flaws we believe we have and become flawless. You only have to look on the front covers of magazines these days to see wrinkles and blemishes air-brushed away. These images show men and women with flawless skin that is totally unrealistic. Yet we as a society have brought into a collective agreement that this is what it means to be beautiful! I am not making a personal judgment about these images as I too have had my share of my photos taken for publications. But the key is to acknowledge that these types of images are not what a person really looks like. To be human *is* to be flawed. There is no beauty in perfection. And if we focus too much attention on our physical selves we cease looking for and see other beautiful parts of ourselves like our souls, and our virtues – the things that make us uniquely who we are in the world. Our flaws are what make us each so unique. And it's our uniqueness that makes us beautiful. In fact, our uniqueness and differences are what we should love about ourselves the most. Consider for a moment if all the flowers in your garden world looked the same . . .

Our first and last love is — self-love.
Christian Bovee (1820–1904)

We all yearn to be loved. But if we want to know *true* love and transform our bodies, we must begin by receiving love from ourselves. You will never find a love greater than the love you can give yourself which ultimately opens the gateway to the greatest love of all – the love from the Universe (God). And from this love of self you not only transform your body and health to be the best they can be, you also become a *giver* of love and spread love wherever you go. The idea that to love oneself is selfish and egotistical is to blindly ignore the real truth about love. Love is not selfish, nor is it egotistical. Love is kind, compassionate, gentle, nurturing, wise, accepting, and powerful. Love is your authentic nature. Love ripples outward when we love ourselves. We can do all things though love. Love is the answer to everything!

The snow goose need not bathe to make itself white. Neither need you do anything but be yourself.
Lao Tzu

Love Will Transform You

Love is the key to your transformation and the healing place for all self-esteem, weight-related issues and difficulties. Love and forgiveness heal our emotional suffering and free us to live fearlessly, passionately and to take care of our health.

When we can reach this place of loving awareness within ourselves, and when we know with certainty we are loved without condition and supported at all times in spite of what we do or don't do, fear stops motivating our behaviors, and we transform. We move forward in our lives by embarking on a journey of grace—a journey of unlimited possibility and potentiality.

When loving becomes your primary way of *being* in the world, it will ripple outward from your hearts into every facet of your life and you find yourself exercising in love, eating in love, drinking in love, having sex in love, connecting in love, working in love—everything!

Love Moves Mountains

When you decide to let love guide your life, the problems that used to feel like mountains will shrink to tiny molehills that you can navigate with ease and grace. Challenges with your weight will no longer have the power they once had. When love fills your entire being, you will cease trying to change your life on the outside and instead focus more on the *inside*. You will enjoy moments of stillness, quiet, and oneness. You take time to sit with your creator and feel grateful. You will appreciate life and all that it affords you, and you make the most of every moment you can. You will think loving thoughts, you will hold loving beliefs, and you will engage in loving behaviors.

Love will transform you.

Love Changes Our Perspective

Love dramatically alters the way we see and express ourselves in the world. Knowing we are loved liberates us to be transparent and to live the truth of who we are without fear. Love lets us experience the company of others as they are without feeling personally affected. Love inspires us to eat foods that have not been tortured or genetically modified and bring harm and disease to our bodies. Love inspires us to regularly move, stretch, and rest our bodies.

When love is absent from a person's life, their view of themselves gets distorted. They cannot see the beauty of themselves, and this casts a dark shadow on the world around them.

There's No Life without Love

When love is absent, we treat ourselves in unloving ways. We do things like criticize our bodies and punish ourselves mentally, emotionally, and physically by engaging in behaviors we know don't serve us—like eating a giant-size popcorn at the movies, when we (here it comes) *should* have bought the smallest size or exercising obsessively in hopes to achieve the 'perfect' physique. We feed our spirit daily with a host of limiting thoughts and beliefs like: *my stomach is gross,*

I'm so stupid because I cry all the time, and *I am fat and ugly.* We stop *listening* to our bodies when we're absent of love and accept that it's reasonable to be carrying around one hundred pounds of unhealthy fat on our body, continue cramming our bodies full of junk, or letting them nearly starve to death.

When love is nowhere in sight, we view ourselves and the world through a harsh and critical lens. We find we are quick to judge and criticize, and we sabotage opportunities to improve our health and lives—like not showing up for your workout when you can't afford not to.

Without love, we fail to see the truth of our magnificence and instead only see the limited identification of self that we continue to hold in place about ourselves through our stories, beliefs, and perceptions. We live in fear, not joy, and anxiety and depression instead of peace. And when love is not present, we look for love in the wrong places. Usually the kitchen, but also in our relationships—and then when the love we need doesn't get fulfilled, we are left feeling disappointed and empty.

Unconditional Love Is the Only True Love

At the root of your physical challenges is a lack of unconditional love and acceptance for who you are. Simplistic as this may sound, it is a beautiful truth, and I invite you to accept it. You can't expect to transform your body if you're not willing to love who you are *now,* as you are now. If you don't find a way to love yourself now, when you lose the weight you feel so unhappy about, it will only be a matter of time before you return to your self-loathing and put the weight back on. It's not always easy to love yourself unconditionally, but it is necessary to begin to try if you want to change your relationship with food and ultimately transform your body. Start by focusing on just one or two things you love, remind yourself of these things daily and build your list from here. Everyone can think of at least of one to two things they love about themselves. And if you get stuck, maybe ask a friend or a loved one to share what it is they love about you. The other day my son said "I love you mom, because you're a funny mom and you play silly." So I add that to my love bank as it wasn't something I had really considered, and now I love that about myself too.

I counseled a woman many years ago who was so in need of unconditional love that during one of her sessions I intuitively felt the need to stop talking, end the session, and just hug this woman with all the love that I could. I held her tight, like I would a small child, and I told her she was safe and loved. She fought me at first, but eventually relaxed and sobbed like a little girl inside my arms. She later told me it was the first time in her entire life she had ever felt loved for no real reason. She told me my loving her was so uncomfortable at first she wanted to hit me and run screaming out of my office. But once she let go and stopped resisting, she said the feeling she felt was indescribable.

So many children are not supported and acknowledged for just *being who they are.* Many children grow up with little or no affection. Lots of children aren't told they're loved or held and hugged "just because." These little people grow up to be big people believing in the false idea that they are loved only under certain conditions, if they believe they are loved at all. Love for many children gets handed out when they do something well at school, are behaving as their parents expect them to behave, or when they are sick or in some kind of pain—although this isn't always the case. But when these children misbehave, or attempt to show up differently in life than their parents, many parents will whip their expressions of love away from their children faster than the speed of light. As a society we do this too. We love you until you fall off the pedestal we have created for you and then we don't love you the same anymore.

Without being aware of it consciously, these children apply the conditions under which they grew up to the ways in which they love themselves. Then, unless they experience a transformation, they will do the same to their children when they have them. Thus the cycle repeats itself, and the idea that love is conditional is handed down from one generation to the next.

Human love is conditional. Divine love has no conditions.

You Are Loved as You Are

Unconditional means *no matter what*. And *you* are loved no matter what you have done, are doing right now, or are going to be doing in the future. Despite what you may have come to believe, you are loved beyond measure and just for being you. You don't have to do or be anything to be loved. All love invites you to do is to love yourself in the same manner and just be true to you. Learn to love yourself unconditionally, and the ability to love others in the same way will become natural—if this is something you want.

When love fills our hearts, we let go of fear and we trust in the natural order and flow of life. Where challenges like exercising regularly and planning healthy meals once felt like an extremely challenging chore, they now feel like easy tasks to accomplish—as simple as brushing your teeth. There are no pre-requisites to being loved—you are loved for simply being you.

If you have a child, think about how much you love your child and how, no matter what they do, your love for them will remain forever constant. Now turn this love toward yourself. If you don't have a child, think about someone you love deeply and then turn the love toward yourself and notice what happens next.

Divine Love

I am very aware that some religious fundamentalists teach that you are not loved unconditionally, and that to be loved you have to follow a specific set of rules. These fundamentalist teachings tell us that Spirit's love for us is conditional and dependent on our behaviors. They say God judges us and deals out retribution when we die and stand before Him. Then, depending on whether you were good or bad, God determines whether you get entry into a blissful heaven or get tossed into fiery hell. They say we should all be "God-fearing," and that *this* is the pathway to your salvation. But these fundamentalists preach a terrible lie that is a huge disrespect to God. What God wants is for you to know you are already loved and to receive the love that available for you. God knows that when you can receive love and you can love yourself this will have a positive effect on everything and everyone around you.

Barriers to Love

Now we can come full circle. At the beginning of chapter 5, I said that if we struggle with our weight, we very likely have been suppressing certain root-cause emotions connected to the fear of rejection and the fear of vulnerability. Very often these root-cause emotions are *shame* and *guilt*. Shame and guilt are big barriers to love, as they are associated with a deep fear of being rejected again. Shame is the idea that we are somehow "bad" or not worthy of love. But this could not be farther from the truth. You have nothing to be ashamed about, nor do you need to feel guilty. If you feel these things, it only tells me that more love is exactly what you need. Shame has a way of not letting us reveal the truth about ourselves for fear we will not be loved. Shame can fuel the belief that vulnerability is weakness, and people who feel shame will do all that they can to not be vulnerable. But vulnerability is in fact *strength*. And only through vulnerability can we let the love we badly need and want back into our hearts.

THOUGHT PROVOKERS

- *What do you see and say to yourself when you look in the mirror?*
- *Do you feel loved just as you are, or do you believe you have to become something more and be a better you first?*
- *Do you act out of a state of love or fear in your life?*
- *Do you trust what your heart tells you, and then do you follow it?*
- *Do you speak kindly to yourself and nurture yourself with tender loving care?*
- *Do you listen to that inner loving voice inside you when it speaks to you?*
- *Do you lovingly acknowledge and release your emotions?*
- *Do you bring love to your suffering, or do you abandon yourself?*
- *Do you eat with love and love what you eat?*
- *Do you lovingly take care of your body?*
- *Do you walk away from toxic people and environments?*
- *Do you look for love in all the wrong places?*

My Reader, You Are Loved!

I don't know any other way to convey this to you right now except through the words on this page and the energy I am pouring from my heart into them.

You are loved! It is okay that you have stopped taking care of yourself. It's okay that you eat four packets of cookies in one sitting because you don't know how to cope differently with your emotional pain. You are flawed—like we all are—and it's okay to love yourself and treat yourself with kindness and compassion. It's okay to surrender and trust and have faith in the unknown. It's okay to feel afraid, and it's okay to feel confused, frustrated, feel helpless and angry. It is all okay. You are loved in spite of your thoughts and feelings. When you can accept everything about yourself, you will set yourself free.

Practices: Self-Love

31 Ways to Love Yourself

Below are 31 beautiful ways for you to begin receiving more love. Begin today. Pick one or two for now and gradually add a few more every few days.

- ❤ Talk to yourself in loving and kind ways. Be aware of critical and judgmental thoughts: instead of believing them and entertaining their presence with your attention, love them and ask them to leave.
- ❤ Give up expectations about who you should and shouldn't be. Focus every minute of every day just being who you are in that moment.
- ❤ Send yourself loving texts.
- ❤ Write out a list of positive affirmations and thoughts about yourself, and then record them and play them back to yourself while driving in your car or out walking or running. For instance, "You are compassionate and kind." "You are a great friend and an excellent mother." "You are thoughtful and considerate." Etc.
- ❤ Invite the universe/God to fill you with love and request that the universe/God assist you in clearing all inner barriers to receiving its love.

- ❤ When you make mistakes and fall off the exercise-and-eating wagon, don't berate yourself. Talk to yourself with kind and encouraging words and invite yourself lovingly to get back on the wagon. Say things to yourself like: "It's okay—so you missed a few days of healthy eating, and you skipped an exercise class in the gym. We will learn from this and discover why we got distracted and get back on track. I love you."

- ❤ Spend time going inward to discover what you are passionate about. Then bring your passions into your daily life. Acknowledging and doing what we are passionate about is an excellent way to show yourself love and respect.

- ❤ During your meditation, send prayers, love, and blessings to others in your life. The more love that you give from within you, the more love will arise from within you.

- ❤ Twice a day, stop and give thanks for your amazing life. Pick at least three things in your life you are grateful for. Gratitude stems from love and creates love.

- ❤ Take the time to regularly ask yourself what you want in life. What do you value? What brings you joy? Then set the intention to bring more of these things into your life.

- ❤ Once a day or whenever you feel like it, whisper the words, "Thank you, God, for loving me."

- ❤ Do loving things for others. Perform random acts of kindness. Remain anonymous and bask privately in the glory of the love you just gave.

- ❤ Listen to your inner voice. Nobody knows you better than you. Take time to go within and connect with yourself.

- ❤ Trust your intuition and follow your heart. Be aware of the messages in your heart and do what *feels* right within you, not what you *think* is right.

- ❤ Remove yourself from toxic people and toxic environments. Send them love and walk away.

- ❤ When you find yourself sending unconditional love to people in your life, such as your children or your clients, be sure to turn that love back on yourself.

- Trust that you are exactly where you are meant to be in life, and remind yourself regularly that you don't need to become anything to be loved.

- Listen to music that opens up your heart and fills you with joy.

- Engage in hobbies, rituals, and activities that open up your heart and bring you joy.

- Be authentic and transparent with the people in your life. You don't have to be anybody other than who you are for the purpose of protecting someone else's feelings.

- Meditate and visualize a ball of light filled with love entering your heart and expanding like the rays of the sun to fill your entire body, and then radiate outward to wrap around the world and every living being in it.

- Write yourself loving notes and affirming messages and post all over your house, car, and workplace.

- Take care of your physical body. Loving ourselves means treating ourselves with kindness and fueling our bodies with the food it needs to be its best.

- Regularly forgive yourself and others (see chapter 7). Forgiveness lets hatred and resentment out and love and kindness in.

- Exercise regularly; move and stretch your body. *Listen* to your body's physical cues and needs, and honor your body by giving it your regular attention.

- Meditate daily to quiet your mind. Go within and *feel* God's eternal love for you.

- Slow down your life and remove unnecessary stressors.

- Several times a day, send love to every cell in your body.

- Be honest with yourself about your feelings. Express them out loud and write them in your journal. Love what arises emotionally and then release it as discussed in chapter 5.

- Keep a journal beside your bed solely for writing down what you love about you, or what I call an I LOVE ME™ journal. Each night before you go to sleep, record in your journal what you love about yourself, what you did that day that you loved, and where in your life you can give yourself more love.

❤ Read the affirmation below at least once a day.

Michelle's Daily Love Affirmation

At the core of who I am is love.
I allow this love to fill me and overflow.
The love I am is endless, and it fuels me day and night.
All that I am is love—endless, unconditional, beautiful, divine love.
I drink regularly from my well of love.
I take excellent care of myself because I love myself.
I am deeply grateful for the love that I am.
I love the love that is God inside me.
God loves me and accepts me just as I am.
I love and accept me just as I am.
I seek only to do that which love invites of me.
I regularly ask myself, "What would love do? What would love say?"
I trust myself implicitly.
I release my emotions and love what is.
I love myself and all that love is.
I fill every space I occupy with my endless supply of love.
Being love brings me joy, and in this joy and love I serve others.
I radiate love.
I love myself and others without expectations.
I live in the present moment where I know love lives.
I glory in who I am.
I am grateful.
My body is a gift. I am a gift.
I love who I am.
I love that I am love.

Through Love's Eyes

As we discovered earlier in the chapter, when we look in the mirror, many of us compartmentalize our bodies: we see ourselves as a flabby arm, a thick thigh, a soft tummy, or a big bum, instead of a whole person. This is a limiting way to view ourselves and the next process will help you see yourself as a whole being, body and soul!

In order to receive the greatest benefit from this process, please do not read ahead. Before you begin, make sure you have about thirty minutes to an hour of uninterrupted privacy and a full-length mirror to stand in front of. Wear a comfortable outfit that reveals your body: a tank top and shorts, bra and underwear, bathing suit, or form-fitting workout clothing. If you feel comfortable doing so, you may also perform this exercise naked.

If you would prefer me to guide you through this process, please go to my website at www.michellearmstrong.com/transformbook and download the audio file "Mirror, Mirror," and I will walk you through each step of the process.

If you would like to follow the process as it's written here, please read and follow each step in sequence:

1. Stand in a relaxed pose facing your full-length mirror. Gently focus on your reflection so that any noises you may be aware of fade into the background. As you look at yourself in the mirror, allow your gaze to move slowly and thoroughly over your entire body. Out loud or silently, describe yourself physically and describe how you feel about what you see. When you feel you are done, go to step 2.

2. How thoroughly have you described yourself? Do you see yourself as attractive, fat, wrinkly, old, young, sexy, big-breasted, flat-chested, too fair, too dark, or just right? Is your hair thick or thin, curly, frizzy, or straight? Do you have love handles, or flab on your upper arms or bicep muscles? Do you see stretch marks or dimples or rolls? Does looking at your body make you feel sick, ashamed, or indifferent? Do you want to cry or laugh? Do you feel disgusted or proud? If there is anything you want to add to your description of yourself, do so now.

3. What else do you see when you look in the mirror? Describe what you see about your personality or character. For example, do you see a sad, depressed person, or an anxious, intense person? Are you person of integrity, or are you holding onto secrets? Are you fearful or brave; are you lazy or a workaholic? Are you addicted to food, sex, booze, or drugs? Do you feel like you need various medications to get through the day? Are you healthy? Do you worry about dying young? Do you consider yourself to be a good mother, sister, daughter, friend, or wife? Do you like sex? Are you happy in your relationship? Do you fantasize about other sexual partners? Are you gay, straight, or bisexual? Are you out? Do you long for a different life, or are you happy where you are? You get the idea.

4. Pick one of your characteristics and locate the places in your body you feel it or see it. If you see yourself as a sad person, do you feel that sadness in your heart or stomach, or do you see it in your eyes? What color is this sadness? Is it blue or gray or lime green? Is the color vibrant or dull? Think of some of the other characteristics and qualities you see in yourself, and go through this process with each one.

5. This is often a very emotional experience. If you feel like crying or laughing or sitting down, please allow yourself to experience your feelings. You are coming to terms out loud with the way you see yourself. This exercise invites you to see the Truth.

6. Are you aware that this is what you think of yourself, say to yourself, and feel about yourself? Are you at all surprised or shocked by the negative image you have of yourself? Is there anything you feel pleased about? For the time being, I'd like you to focus exclusively on the negative ways in which you see yourself. I'd like you to call to mind your children, your significant other, or dearest friend—anyone you love unconditionally. If you can think of no one in your life at the moment, is there a beloved animal or someone from your past you love or loved unconditionally? When you think of this loved one, what types of words come to mind? Do you think of the loved one as beautiful, darling, dear, sweet, charming, wonderful, or adorable? Would you ever speak to your beloved sister or

son or dog the way you speak to yourself? Why not? Do you agree that you'd probably never speak to any other human being the way you speak to yourself?

7. Would you like to see yourself as you truly are? If your answer is yes, I will ask you now, for the purpose of this exercise, to open your mind and heart to the idea that there is something greater than yourself operating out in the universe. Think of this energy as all-encompassing, unconditionally loving, and available to you right now and always. Perhaps you believe in God or a divine presence or a higher power of some kind. If you don't or you're not sure, can you think of this energy as Love?

Focus on this energy now, whether it is the spirit of a deceased Loved One, God, Goddess, the Universe, Soul, Buddha, Christ, Allah, Krishna, Zeus, Archangel Michael, Mother Mary, Nature, Infinity, Light, Love, or anything that resonates for you.

Read step 8 several times until you feel you can recall it easily. You will be guiding yourself through this process with your eyes closed. Still facing the mirror, take a couple of deep, cleansing breaths, relax your body (you may sit down if you want), close your eyes, and take yourself through the process.

8. Now that you have identified the source of the greatest love you can imagine, invite that energy into your body. Imagine that the energy enters through the top of your head and goes down through your body, through your shoulders, chest, abdomen, hips, and into your feet. This is the White Light of Pure Love entering into your body. Stay with this feeling for a moment.

Now, go ahead and release all the negative thoughts you have about yourself to this White Light. Take all the judgments you have about yourself—all that you have now, and all that you've had in the past—gather them all up, and pass them over to that energy. Take all your beliefs about what life should be like, and also hand them over to the Light. Take all your memories, from the long-ago past, from when you were a teenager, from yesterday—any memory associated with the way you think about yourself today—and hand them over as well.

I want you to allow that energy to fully permeate your being. Allow Love's thoughts and beliefs to enter. It's okay if you don't even know what they are—just invite them into your Being. Imagine Love rising from your feet all the way up through your knees, hips, chest, shoulders, and up through the top of your head.

Now I'm going to invite you to do something you've never done before. I'm going to invite you to see yourself through the eyes of Pure Love. You no longer hold those other filters—your limiting beliefs, your negative self-image, your damning judgments, or your painful memories. You have handed them over. In your own time, open your eyes, and you will be seeing yourself for the first time as you truly are—through the eyes of Pure Love.

9. Standing now, with your eyes open, look at yourself in the mirror and again describe everything you see and feel.

10. What do you see now? Do you see Beauty, Light, Love, God, and Perfection? Do you see that you are perfectly you, exactly as you are meant to be? As you continue looking in the mirror through the eyes of Pure Love, how do you feel about the unkind things you used to say to yourself? Do you still see those things? My guess is that you see only the Beauty, Truth, Light, and Love that you have always been and will always be!

I see you as you truly are: perfect, gorgeous, magnificent, and divine!

11. Treat your beautiful self to a luxurious bath, a peaceful walk in nature, or a cuddle with your children or beloved. Be kind to yourself—you are precious and loved always!

CHAPTER 7
FORGIVENESS

The tragedy of life is not death, but what
we let die inside us while we live.
Norman Cousins

When I was in my teens, I was raped at a house party by a boy I knew. I had a very low self-image back then, and when that happened, it compounded my feelings of self-hatred. For years and years I kept this experience a secret because of the shame and guilt I felt about it. I binge drank and binge ate, and I smoked cigarettes—all as a way to cope with my internal suffering, which eventually resulted in depression. The story I repeatedly told myself was that it was somewhat my fault because I'd been drinking. I repeatedly imposed judgment and blame on myself: *I should have known better—I'm so stupid.*

When I finally decided to let go of this story and the pain that surrounded this experience, I knew my next step was forgiveness. I needed not to just forgive the boy, I needed to forgive *myself* for all the damaging ways I'd tortured myself mentally and physically, and for blaming myself for what had happened. As soon as I forgave, I experienced relief, and the enormous emotional burden I carried was lifted.

As I went through my forgiveness process, I completely *surrendered*. In other words, I accepted "what is" and let go of the expectations I had of life and myself. In this surrendering, I discovered a love inside me that was eternal and immense enough to allow me to love both myself and the boy who raped me. I realized that it was actually because of a lack of love we both had for ourselves that this boy and I found ourselves in the situation we did.

The gateway to healing is Love.

Now, don't misunderstand me. I'm not excusing rape. It is never okay to abuse or harm another living being. All I am suggesting is that there are reasons for why things happen, and that the true source of hatred and evil is not hatred and evil. Hatred and evil are symptoms of a lack of love. Also, if that boy hadn't done what he had done to me, I would not be who I am today. As strange as it might sound to someone still suffering in hurt, I am *grateful* for that experience, because of what it has taught me and invited me to become in my life. But only through a genuine and heartfelt desire to forgive, coupled with a deep love and desire to heal, can we recognize the truth of this reality.

Forgiveness is the fragrance the violet shed on the heel that crushed it.

Mark Twain

Forgiveness Isn't Always Easy, but It Is Always Necessary

To return to the process we began in chapter 5, to fully release your suppressed emotions, the next step in your healing journey is to open your heart and forgive. You cannot fully release the pain and suffering you feel inside without walking the pathway of forgiveness, and you will not be able to permanently transform your body until you have healed emotionally. If, as you went through the practices in the previous chapter, you found that there were some emotional experiences you just couldn't embrace and release, then forgiveness is what beckons you next. *Listen to what your inner voice is telling you.*

Forgiveness is not something we do—it's who we are.

Rhonda's Story

When I first met Rhonda, she was about twenty-five pounds overweight. Rhonda was twenty-nine at the time and owned her own graphics design business. She was smart and attractive, but lacked confidence in herself big time. Rhonda initially came to see me for some life purpose coaching. Once we got into Rhonda's story, it became quickly apparent that Rhonda had a wealth of anger and resentment inside her toward her mother, whom she described as "critical, disrespectful, and interfering." She told me about some of things her mother had done, and she was right—her mother seemed just as she described. However, the issue at hand was not her mother's *behavior*, but rather Rhonda's suppressed rage at her mother. It was Rhonda's rage that was triggering her to eat and gain weight.

For almost a year I worked with Rhonda, gently encouraging her to forgive her mother and see her mother in a new light. I helped her set some healthy boundaries and let go of the expectations *she* had created for her mother.

For almost a year Rhonda resisted forgiveness like crazy—until the day came when the feelings of rage she felt inside became greater than her resistance to forgiving. Her rage was literally consuming her, and she knew she needed to address it if she wanted her body and her life to change.

When Rhonda finally forgave her mom, she, like many of us do, wished she had done so much sooner. Through the healing power and beauty of forgiveness, Rhonda was able to see her mother in a totally new way—one that made her realize her mother's behaviors had nothing to do with her. Her mother was simply doing the best she could based on her childhood programming and understanding.

Rhonda then forgave herself for inviting so much rage into her heart and her body, and she lovingly began forgiving herself when she didn't always show up *perfectly*—which, by the way, nobody does.

Rhonda and her mom didn't end up being best friends as a result of her forgiveness, but Rhonda's life transformed, and what do you know? She started to lose her weight.

When we forgive and free ourselves from suffering, we become the person we want to be.

Why Is It So Hard to Forgive?

One primary reason people resist forgiveness is that forgiveness requires the feelings of deep hurt and sadness beneath their anger and resentment to surface, and they are afraid of what it will mean to let go of these feelings. The other barrier to forgiveness is simply that people don't want to forgive and would rather hold on to their anger and resentments. These people have stories and beliefs, like: *There's no way I'm going to allow myself to be hurt by them again—NO WAY!"* and *Forgiveness is weakness. I hate weakness, and it just means the people who hurt me don't suffer at all for all the pain and heartache they caused me. They don't deserve my forgiveness? Forget it!*

But it's important to realize that these ideas and beliefs are just *stories*. They're stories you've used as a protective mechanism to keep yourself emotionally safe—but also trapped. They're stories you have created and perpetuated that serve only to keep you stuck inside a body that limits your true potential but what you have come to believe is some form of self-preservation.

But you cannot be free to be who you want to be with limiting stories and beliefs like these. If you really want to change and transform, you need to choose new and empowering stories (see Chapter 1) and be willing to face the emotional pain beneath the anger and forgive, with the understanding and foresight that doing so benefits *you,* not the person or persons who harmed you. They don't need to know you've forgiven them (unless you want them to). Forgiveness is not for anyone else—it's something you do for *yourself.*

To forgive is to set a prisoner free and then realize that prisoner was you.

Lewis Smedes

When people inflict pain on another, it is *always* because of the lack of love they have for themselves. People in *love* do not harm, hurt, or condemn. And when people can come to the awareness of this truth, they can have compassion and understanding for why others hurt us and why we at times hurt others too as well as ourselves. Eating food you know is unhealthy for your body is a way you abuse and inflict harm on yourself. Telling yourself, once you've eaten the unhealthy food, what a worthless piece of nothingness you are, is another way of inflicting self-harm.

Forgiveness is not a one-time act. It's a habit that becomes who you are.

An Eye for an Eye—How's That Working for You?

While there often arises a strong desire within us when we've been hurt to punish and harm those responsible (i.e., "an eye for an eye"), this way of thinking does not allow for any healing, transformation, or growth. You can condemn and hold rage till the cows come home, but the emotional suffering you feel inside will not leave you. It will stay in your body and continue to fester. It will continue to limit your life and potential. If anything, this way of thinking serves only to perpetuate and give power to limiting emotional experiences, such as rage, anger, and resentment. Then you become formed from the same emotional mold that hurt you in the first place. Is this really what you want?

Condemning Doesn't Fix the Problem of Pain: Love and Forgiveness Do

One day I hope all of humanity will understand the damage that is done when we put our criminals in cages without taking their stories into account. I hope that we will come to realize that every criminal has a story of pain and suffering (just like you) that got them to the place they now are, and take the time to assist them in healing emotionally instead of condemning them to eternal (and temporal) hell. But this is a matter of personal opinion. I'm not here to judge or preach. I only share my personal vision about forgiveness with you because I *know* the gift forgiveness and love can bring.

When we resist forgiveness, we put our heart in a cage, and then throw away the key to our life. When we choose instead to forgive ourselves and others, we liberate our hearts from suffering.

Set Yourself Free

The willingness to forgive takes deep resolve and a fully open heart, which is why it is such a powerful, healing process. As you forgive all the people in your past and present for all the ways you feel they hurt or harmed you (or continue to hurt and harm you), your heart will expand, and the love you feel inside of you will have a ripple effect through your behaviors and all aspects of your life. Instead of torturing yourself verbally and condemning yourself in your mind when you eat two more slices of pizza than you'd intended *(Well, I've done it now; I might as well eat a tub of ice cream, too.)*, you'll forgive yourself, love yourself, and move on. And because self-love truly is the key to transforming yourself from the inside out, the next time might find yourself behaving differently.

Forgiveness cannot change your past, but it can certainly alter your future.

Forgiveness Heals

I cannot overstate the power of forgiveness in your inward journey toward transformation, especially if you have any stubborn emotional blocks remaining after completing the practices in chapters 5 and 6. Forgiveness is your gateway to emotional freedom and healing your issues with your body for good. The act of forgiving creates a beautiful and powerful opportunity to surrender your anger, resentments, and frustrations, and lift the burden of your emotional discomfort so you can powerfully move in the direction of health and wellness, live the life you want, and be the person you desire to be. Forgiveness removes negative energy in relationships—especially the relationship we have with ourselves! When we forgive ourselves or someone else, we let the pain and suffering go, and a beautiful space gets created within us that automatically fills us up with deep and rich love, compassion, acceptance, and understanding—all the things we *need* to feel if we want to heal and transform our bodies.

Forgiveness Allows for Love and Peace

Through forgiving others, you will come to know yourself as the courageous, loving, and fearless person you are. And, even more importantly, you will forgive yourself for all the ways you have harmed and hurt yourself (and I suspect you are still hurting yourself now).

When my clients and I regularly forgive, we feel an immediate sense of lightness, love, connectedness, and joy fill our spirits. When audience members at my workshops experience forgiveness, a feeling of lightness fills them also, and they actually look different in appearance. The dark heaviness within them lifts. I can literally see light surrounding them. They seem to radiate with a beautiful softness and strength that dissolves the dark cloud they once carried in their bodies.

After a session of forgiveness with private clients, I often encourage them to look at themselves in the mirror. I want them to see what I can see—their true beauty, grace, lightness, and divinity.

Forgiveness is a divine tool through which we can regularly cleanse and heal all of human suffering. By making forgiveness a daily ritual, you will avoid getting dragged down into the low emotional vibrations that trigger you to binge-eat and pin your butt to the couch instead of taking it for a walk.

When you can make forgiveness a part of who you are, it becomes easier and easier to maintain empowering states such as love, peace, and joy, which are the emotional and energetic states you need in order to know when you've have enough to eat, what is best for you to eat, when you need to move, stretch, and strengthen your body, and when you need to go within.

In my entire life, I have not met a single person who did not want love, joy, and peace in his or her life. This is because we know this to be who we really are—our authentic nature and the place from which we have all come. Without all the emotional baggage, love, peace, and joy are our true essence, refracted vibrantly through our unique personalities.

The commonly held belief that someone or something outside ourselves inflicts pain and suffering *on* us is a disempowering perception. All pain and suffering arises from within—via our beliefs, our stories, our mental interpretations, and our ongoing decisions to continue harboring feelings of anger and resentment because we are afraid to feel our truth. In this instance, suffering is a choice. If we choose instead to forgive, then we are also choosing to put an end to our suffering and to live a better life.

Those who turn away from the light will spend their life in the darkness.

Forgiveness Is a Choice

While it may feel like every fiber of your being wants to cling to its feelings of hatred, resentment, and revenge, you must rise above your ego and pride if you want to release your emotional baggage and set your soul free. Believe me, I do know how difficult it can be to forgive, and what a challenge it is to quell that annoying voice inside that says, *Forget them! I'm not forgiving them for what they did to me!*

But you need to understand that this type of egotistical, prideful, and limited thinking is what is keeping you stuck. "They" are not being affected by your withholding; it's you—and only you—who is continuing to suffer.

As I tell my clients and workshop attendees, forgiveness is a choice. It is a willingness to open up your heart and act in blind faith from a deep inner knowing within yourself, to rise above your ego and your pride, to face and release the hurt and pain you know deep within doesn't benefit you.

Forgive them, Father, for they do not know what they do.
Jesus

You have to choose to let your pain go. Forgiveness will free your soul and make it so much easier to lose the fat and transform your body. Your feelings of anger, resentment, rage, and hurt are only harming your body, not benefiting it. And when you free yourself from the burden of these emotions, you'll no longer have to eat to suppress them.

When many ponder forgiveness,
it can be viewed as foolish and weak,
to open one's heart to hurt again,
and turn the other cheek.
But if you look beyond this story,
through your heart and not your mind,
you'll awaken a loving truth within;
"Forgiveness" is what you'll find.
And while surrendering your anger,
means acknowledging your pain,

you know in your heart it must be done,
if you ever wish to feel whole again.
So even though you're hurting,
rise above your ego and pride,
forgive the person who hurt you,
and let love in your heart abide.
I promise when you've done this,
Your heart and soul you'll free,
to become the truth of who you really are,
and fulfill your soul's destiny.

When we are willing to release all our emotional pain and suffering once and for all through forgiveness, we sever the energetic and emotional ties that bind us to an old event, person, or story from our past or present. If we continue to drag this unhappy experience into every moment of our lives, we will continue to suffer needlessly.

My dear reader, you are remarkable, amazing, and a worthy-of-all-things-good human being. You deserve to let go of the hurt you feel inside so you can move on, transform your body, and live an extraordinary life!

Forgive yourself for allowing yourself to continue to be hurt by the past.

Karen's Story

I recently facilitated a forgiveness session with a client named Karen, a thirty-seven-year-old single mom who was battling with her weight and suffering from depression. She needed to forgive her ex-husband, who had cheated on her several times and who then left her for one of the women he was cheating with two days after the birth of their son. Karen was a chronic binge eater and a massive avoider of her feelings. As a result of the pain in her emotional body, she struggled to transform her body, but even though she exercised regularly, her eating habits were counterproductive. She sought emotional comfort and respite from her pain through chocolates, cookies, potato chips, pastries, and ice cream. On many occasions she would clear her kitchen of these foods, just to find herself two days later shopping for these items once again. She saw no other way to free herself from her pain than to eat foods she knew were making her fat and sick.

Karen despised the idea of being vulnerable and would regularly suffer in silence instead of choosing to reach out for help. She felt ashamed and unworthy of kindness and love from others. Karen found it extremely difficult to consider the idea of loving herself. She said the idea of it made her feel sick. But her saving grace was to participate in forgiveness, which arose from the love for her son. While loving herself seemed an impossible task, loving her son was easy and effortless.

So one day I said to Karen, "Anything less than loving yourself isn't really loving your son, now, is it? Because as much as you love your son, he will learn to treat himself the very same way you treat yourself. Your words will fall on deaf ears. He will model your behaviors, not what you say. And he will come to believe what you now do, that to love oneself is unacceptable. He will believe he is not worthy, just as you feel you are not worthy. And no matter how much you love him, it won't make an iota of a difference. Your parents love you, too; am I right? Do you want this experience for your son?"

When she of course said "no," I asked her why, and she said, "Because I love my son and I want him to know he is loved. I don't want him to suffer the emotional pain that I do."

"Oh, I see," I said quietly. "Just so I am hearing you correctly, what you're saying is: it's okay for your *son* to experience unconditional love, but it's not okay for you, is that right?"

I also asked her if she ever stopped loving her son when he was hurt or angry, or when he made mistakes or showed poor judgment. The answer, of course, was, "No, never. I will never stop loving my son."

Again I asked, "But it's okay to stop loving yourself when you are hurt and angry, and when you make mistakes, is this right?" I asked, "Who would you be free to be if you didn't have this hurt and anger? How different would life be for you? How different would it be for your son?"

After some consideration of these questions, Karen agreed to forgive herself.

Forgiving the past allows you to live freely and fearlessly in the present.

Forgiveness Means Living Your Life to Its Fullest!

Remember, forgiveness does not mean we have to accept a person's behaviors. We don't need to accept rape, physical violence, verbal, emotional, or psychological abuse, criticism, lies, and betrayal. But what we can do is forgive the person who engaged in these behaviors through a divine understanding that their behaviors have *nothing* to do with us, and that they were doing the best they could with the resources they had available to them at the time. You were not at fault for the behaviors others chose at the time they were hurtful toward you. Undoubtedly there have been times you have hurt yourself and others, and this same truth applies to you. Each one of us is always doing the best we can with the inner resources we have in that moment, and sometimes, many times, we do selfish and cruel things out of our own suffering.

To err is human, to forgive, divine.
Alexander Pope

It's important to understand that forgiveness is best conducted without any expectations. Forgiveness does not necessarily *change* the other person or their behaviors, and in most cases it doesn't. Changing others is not the purpose of forgiveness. Forgiveness is a self-loving and heartfelt decision to consciously *release* all anger, resentment, guilt, shame, depression, and thoughts of revenge or retaliation. Also, forgiveness does not mean forgetting, or erasing this event from your life. Once you forgive, whatever it was that hurt you so greatly will still be a part of who you are, but it will no longer be at the *center* of who you are. It will no longer control your actions and behaviors or strangle the love in your heart. It will no longer prevent you from loving yourself, taking care of yourself, and being who you want to be.

In addition to the feeling of peace and love that pervades every cell of your being when you forgive, you will also experience a greater ongoing level of psychological and spiritual well-being, healthier relationships, less stress, relief from depression and anxiety, weight loss, and even a decrease in physical pain. Forgiveness has even been shown to lower blood pressure! When you can release all grudges, resentments, and hurts and forgive the person or persons who hurt you, including yourself, the past will no longer define you, and you'll be free to live your life without limits.

Like sky-diving, forgiving can feel scary at first, but once you let go and jump, the wings of love will catch you and liberate you forever from the prison of your hurt. Without a doubt, the hardest thing you'll ever have to do is to forgive. But once it is done, you will realize it was the most empowering and awesome thing you can do, and you'll want to do it again and again. This may be hard to swallow right now, but trust me, it is true.

Forgiveness is more than a feeling; it's a promise not to use the past behavior of others against them ever again.

Jane's Story

When I first met Jane, she was at least one hundred pounds overweight and transparent about the anger and rage she felt toward her mother. She totally blamed her mother for her weight. As a result of the anger she had harbored for many years, Jane had turned to all sorts of different forms of abuse to cope with her *true* feelings behind her anger, which were hurt and abandonment. But for many years before we'd met, Jane simply was not ready to release the hurt and see her mother in any other light than as a "bitch."

When Jane did forgive her mother, she was amazed at how different she felt. Not only did her rage seem to instantly lift, but she was able to see her mother through different eyes and experience the realization that her mother loved her very much and was simply doing the best she could as a result her own childhood programming and life experiences. Jane wished, as many who forgive their parents also do, she could tell her mother how sorry she was for having been so judgmental and for limiting the potential of the relationship they could have had—especially when she also recognized that she herself had made many mistakes as a parent. In Jane's case, she was not able to physically say she was sorry. Jane's mother had passed. So instead she wrote her mom a letter and bawled her eyes out as she did so.

You will know that forgiveness has occurred within you when you think of those who hurt you and you feel a strong desire within to wish them well.
Lewis B. Smedes

In the case of horrific abuse and heinous acts, it may take a lifetime to forgive, but a daily ritual of forgiving will soon begin to erode the anger, hurt, and resentment you feel. (You'll receive practical guidance about developing this ritual in the practices section at the end of the chapter.) Little by little, suffering is lessened. But as we loosen our limiting emotions of fear and anger and embrace the empowering emotions of love and forgiveness, our suffering is replaced with an experience of the divine essence of love within. We become aware that we are free to live the truth of ourselves, and through this love we can once again share our magnificence with the world.

When you hold resentment toward another, you are bound to that person or condition by an emotional link

that is stronger than steel. Forgiveness is the only way to
dissolve that link and be free.
                        Catherine Ponder

Forgiveness is a gift we give to ourselves, and through our forgiving we can come to know a deeper level of love within ourselves and for ourselves and others. Forgiveness is not something we *do* for someone else. It is a practice of healing the pain inside of us so we can experience the life we so ache to experience—a life of health, joy, peace, and love!

Can You Forgive Yourself?

As difficult as it can be to forgive others, perhaps the most difficult person to forgive is yourself. Even those who have no trouble forgiving others and giving others the benefit of the doubt strongly resist forgiving themselves, often because of a deep lack of self-love. But continuing to hold resentment and anger in your heart, *even toward yourself,* is not the way to respond and cope to life's difficulties, nor is it the way to live a healthy and extraordinary life. By holding onto past events that are painful, we keep them alive and flaming.

On many occasions I have witnessed clients begin to cry as they recite the list of all the people they are choosing to forgive. But when I reach the point in my forgiveness process where I invite them to forgive themselves also, there is nearly always a slight moment of hesitation before they collapse in an intense wave of grief. They are grieving for themselves—that they had cut themselves off from love for so long, and that they had stopped treating themselves with kindness and compassion during the most challenging moments in their lives. They realize they stopped loving themselves, and they say, "I'm sorry" over and over again to themselves, until it seems they can say it no more. It is a great moment of transcendence for many and, for me as a witness and teacher of forgiveness, a beautiful reminder of the power of forgiveness and the love and light of the Divine within us all. Forgiveness brings with it divine understanding. It puts the past behind you where it absolutely belongs, so you can freely move forward into the life of your own making.

We see the lessons and gifts inside those old hurtful circumstances, and we recognize that at some level we needed to experience those events in order to become the people we are destined to be in this lifetime. We recognize suffering as an opportunity to spiritually evolve and grow. We come to understand that without those past experiences, we would not be able to be the people we are today. We begin to understand our true potential. We start to view those experiences with an overwhelming sense of gratitude and grace, and we feel appreciative to all the people involved, because we recognize that without them we would not be able to fulfill our destiny to be who we want to be.

Consider a time in your past when you did something hurtful simply because you didn't know any better at the time. Now that you know what you do now, you wouldn't repeat those same behaviors again, would you?

THOUGHT PROVOKERS

- *Who do you know right now that you need to forgive?*
- *How much longer are you prepared to suffer needlessly?*
- *What are you most afraid will happen when you forgive?*
- *How does this fear serve you?*
- *In what ways do you benefit by holding on to your anger and resentments?*
- *Who will you be free to be when you've released the pain you feel?*
- *What do you need to believe in order to forgive and let go?*
- *How did you feel about the stories in this chapter?*
- *Were there aspects of these stories you can relate to?*
- *In what ways do you need to forgive yourself?*

Even after learning about all the benefits of forgiveness, you may still find yourself resisting it. If you are one of these people, I say to you now, from the bottom of my heart, how truly sorry I am that you have suffered to such a degree that you have chosen to close your heart and dim your beautiful light. But I want you to know that living in resentment requires an enormous amount of heavy, negative, and exhausting energy. It is easy for me to spot those fearful and reluctant to forgive. They suffer visibly, wearing their pain in their physical bodies. The pain and resentment they've carried for years are etched upon their faces. There is darkness in their energy field. Life is a constant struggle.

You do not need to continue to live your life this way. Put down the heavy bricks of hurt you are feeling and use the power of forgiveness to free you. My reader: you are an amazing person! So courageous and beautiful—and so wise. I know you know it's the right thing to do. You are strong, and you can handle this. You will not dissolve or fall apart as you think, I promise. You are not weak. You are fearless! It will serve you greatly to love and forgive, and when you are ready, I know in my heart you will do so.

You have to love yourself enough to want your own suffering to end. Decide when you have had enough, then release your past and forgive yourself and all others associated with your suffering so you can move on and heal your body. Look deep inside the vastness of your heart and know and trust that you are loved and safe. Know you are capable of real, lasting forgiveness, and that you *deserve* the benefits you will receive when you forgive.

You have the power to forgive. Forgiveness is your true nature.

Set the Intention to Forgive Now

Now we are going to shift to the practice of forgiveness. To begin, all you need is a heartfelt willingness to seek out the love in your heart for the person whose behaviors hurt you, and to move on and tell a different, more empowering story.

Keep in mind that forgiving others does not necessarily mean that we experience reconciliation with that person or that we must now interact with those who once hurt us. This is not necessary for forgiveness to occur.

Also, forgiveness can be achieved remotely, without ever having to be in contact with that person. Forgiveness can also be accomplished in stages if you are not quite ready to let it all go now. If you'd like to begin slowly, you can begin your forgiveness journey as follows.

- First, decide that you want to forgive and are ready to surrender your anger, and resentments and change your life.
- Second, humble yourself in the awareness that what you've tried up to now hasn't worked.
- Next, set a heartfelt intention (ideally through meditation) to hold in your heart and mind the willingness to forgive and release your hurt and anger.
- Then pray for the courage to forgive. Pray for the strength to see yourself through your emotional releasing. (This is not mandatory for those who don't pray, but it is certainly very effective and for those who do pray I strongly encourage it.)
- Finally, write in a journal and express all the true thoughts and feelings you have around the person/s whom you wish to forgive. Be utterly transparent. The more truthful you can be with yourself, the greater your transformation will be.
- Then when you're ready, engage in the practices below.

Practices: Forgiveness

To move more deeply into your forgiveness journey, I invite you to engage in all of the practices listed below—intuitively selecting whichever one feels right to begin with. You may just choose to do just one practice for now, or all of them—and that's okay. Whatever you choose, trust in your heart that it's the perfect choice for what you need right now to move forward. All is well. You are loved and you are safe.

Write a Forgiveness Letter

Write a letter to the person or persons who hurt you and whom you're allowing through your stories to continue to hurt you. If that person is *you*, then write the letter to you. In your letter, state what hurt you, how it hurt you, and what impact this hurt has had on your life up to now. Refrain from blaming in your letter.

Simply state your feelings using 'I' statements such as, "I feel hurt because…" and be as transparent as you can. Here is an example of how you might begin your letter.

Dear _____,

When you lied to me five years ago about having a relationship with another woman, I felt betrayed and hurt. Since then, I have been unable to open my heart to trust other people, and men in particular. I realize that it was I who chose to close my heart, not you, but because I was hurting so much and because I was so angry with you, I did not know how to manage my feelings any differently. But now I realize that by holding onto my angry feelings toward you, I am preventing myself from moving forward with my life, and I need to let go. I have also realized that I have only been able to see one side of the story, as I do not know what was going on in your life that may have contributed to your behaviors. I forgive you.

Forgiveness Meditation

If you regularly practice meditation, begin your meditation practice as you normally do. If you do not, you can use the Centering Meditation process in the book's introduction. When you have reached a deep place of stillness, visualize the crown of your head opening and a healing light entering it from above, filling every fiber of your being from your head all the way to your toes. Visualize this light surrounding your heart and filling it with love and peace. Invite your Higher Power, the angels, Jesus, Allah, or whatever form of comfort feels right for you, to give you the courage to look deeply within your emotional body. Then scan your emotional body with the intention of seeking out pain, hurts, anger, and resentments, as well as the people or events attached to these emotions. Then, if it feels right at this time to release these emotional energies from your body, simply say to these energies, *"Thank you for being a part of me and for taking such good care of me. But now I wish to move forward in my life, and I lovingly release you back from whence you came. I love you. I thank you. Please leave my body."* Then, when your meditation is complete, journal what came to your awareness and what you experienced.

Find the Gift and Lesson

Inside of every tragedy and hurtful experience is a gift and opportunity to grow that awaits your awareness and acknowledgment. When we choose to *seek out* that gift, we will find it, learn, and then let go. We will come to a divine understanding that this event had to happen this way for you to come to know the truth of *who you really are*. And once you have the awareness of this gift, the pain you felt about it will go away.

Go into a deep meditation and fill your body with the same healing light as described in the Forgiveness Meditation above. Invite your Higher Power, or whatever term you use to denote your Higher Power, to support you in your journey to find the gift that will set you free. Then, in your mind's eye, imagine floating up above your body and then being gently pulled back to that past time and event where you were hurt. Then, with the assumption that this event does hold a gift for you, ask yourself, *What did I want to get from this event that I did not get at that time? What do I need to receive now that will allow me to release my feelings of hurt?* Ask your Higher Power to show you the lesson from this event that will set you free emotionally. Ask yourself, *If indeed there was a positive purpose (gift) and reason (lesson) for this event, what might this gift and lesson be?* Trust that an intuitive answer will arise in you and this answer will set you free. Then express gratitude for this learning experience, and gently and slowly float back along the line of time in your mind, back to the present moment, and open your eyes. Journal your thoughts and experiences.

CHAPTER 8

BEYOND FEAR

There is nothing to be afraid of in life—not even fear itself.

When I was in my early twenties, I decided to face my fears through an experience. What better way to achieve this intention than to leap out of an airplane ten thousand feet in the air (wearing a parachute, of course!). Since I had a lot of fears about, well, pretty much everything, strapping myself to a total stranger and leaping into a vast space of nothingness seemed very apropos.

As the plane began its ascent and we climbed up into the sky, I sat harnessed to the front of a stranger whom I silently prayed was an experienced jumper who would not let me fall. I felt the fear rising within as my ego-mind screamed at me like I had lost my mind: *Stop this ridiculous nonsense now and get the heck out of Dodge!* Perhaps I was losing my mind, but my soul foresaw that something greater was about to happen—and it was leaping up and down inside of me like my four-year-old set loose in a Toys 'R Us® store. Somewhere in the depths of my awareness, I knew I needed to face and move beyond everything I'd come to fear in my life if I wanted to discover something deeper and more profound about myself—even if it meant leaping with blind faith into the unknown.

As I stared out the gaping hole of the small Cessna aircraft, out of which I'd soon be tumbling and then falling at a speed of approximately 200 kilometers per hour toward earth, I experienced a momentary panic attack. The following thought arose in my head: *I can't do this! What am I doing?! I'm going to die!* But this thought disappeared as quickly as it arose. I was done with the way I'd been living my life, and I was tired of giving my fears so much control. I knew the time had come to move beyond my fears, and I knew there was no turning back. *I'm doing this,* I said back to the thought through committed, gritted teeth, *and this time you're not going to stop me.*

My jumping partner tapped me on the shoulder. "On the count of three, we jump!" he yelled through the loud noise of the aircraft engines. I craned my neck to look back at the stranger I'd known for less than an hour and acknowledged to myself that I was placing my life in his hands—my heart seem to cease beating. He looked me square in the eye and asked me a question I knew had a double meaning: "ARE YOU READY TO JUMP?"

Are *you* ready to face your fears?

The Time Has Come

I invite you now to welcome and embrace your fears. Only when we know what's at the center of our fears can we then *use* our fears to propel us into the life and body we've always wanted and known in hearts in our ultimate destiny and truth. While your fears can seem intensely real, they are really nothing more than illusions created by your ego-mind as a form of self-protection. They were created at a time in your life when you experienced some form of intense emotional suffering—when you forgot the eternal nature of your being in that you are always safe and loved beyond measure. When we can move beyond our fears and step into the awareness of what's on the other side (i.e., our truth), we will come to see that our fears are really teachers in disguise and opportunities to learn something greater about ourselves we hadn't previously known. In fact, we realize, through the pathways of truth and awareness, that our fears themselves are not real in and of themselves, but stories we've come to believe. We also arrive at what's on the other side of fear, which is limitless and abundant Love.

THOUGHT PROVOKER
- *What are you afraid of?*

Our Greatest Fear

Often, when I invite a client to go within and investigate their emotional body, the response is often one of intense fear—not unlike the scene in horror movies where the barefoot woman wearing a nightgown is walking on tip-toe down her hallway, breathing shallowly, with her eyes wide, a kitchen knife in her hand, preparing to attack or flee. She knows something is out there that just isn't right; she just doesn't know what it is. Her mind starts playing its little tricks and feeds her all sorts of ideas and telling her stories that are fueling and heightening her terror. She fears whatever might be around the corner. She is afraid of the *unknown*.

> *Fear is not something we need to be afraid of, as fear itself holds no power. The fastest way to eliminate fear is to remind yourself you are safe and loved and to breathe slowly and deeply.*

This fear of self-inquiry is so scary for many people, that they carve out a particular groove in their lives, one they are familiar with, and then rarely deviate from this groove even if makes them unhappy—all to avoid having to face their fears. As much as a woman may want to leave her abusive husband, she will often stay because of what she has conditioned herself to believe through her stories and because she feels safer with the devil she knows. The unknown just seems too terrifying. Yet the unknown is what holds the gift of transformation and freedom.

Whenever I invite my clients to pause for few seconds and go within themselves *before* reaching for the second piece of cake or handful of cookies, it evokes feelings of discomfort and uncertainty which are symptoms of a much bigger fear which is the truth of what's really going on, surfacing to get their attention and awareness. While they are not aware of it in at the time, what they're afraid of is their own extinction. Since they so strongly identify with the stories that are intertwined with their fears, they intuitively sense an existential crisis is imminent as it becomes clear that the truth of these stories must cease to exist for the truth of who they truly are to surface. And because they don't know what this truth is, they feel as though it's something *unknown* and it evokes fear and *panic*. Yet when we have faith that the fear isn't real and that it's only the *story* that dies, and trust that we don't die, we can release the need to panic, walk fearlessly into the center of our fears and transform them from the inside out.

> *Death is our greatest fear, because we believe that in death we die. But that is not true. It is only our physical bodies that die. The truth of who we are, which is our Awareness and our consciousness, remains intact and eternal.*

Fiona's Story

When I met Fiona, she was 45, married with children, and a very successful entrepreneur. She owned her own business and was doing extremely well financially. Fiona came to see me because she had an intense fear of "not having any money" and admitted that she believed there was a "possibility" in the very near future that she could lose some of the money she'd been storing away like a squirrel for her future. Fiona was also overweight and found it difficult to eat healthy food. Whenever her fears of not having money would arise, Fiona would eat something sugary—her "food cocaine."

Fiona came from a broken and dysfunctional home so she moved out when she was only fourteen. She didn't have a penny to rub together at that time and had to make her own way in the world. Within ten years Fiona had become a millionaire.

After hearing Fiona's story and her concern about "not having any money," I invited Fiona to dig a little deeper by asking her to repeat after me, "If I have no money, I am afraid . . ." She said, "If I have no money, I am afraid I will become a bag lady on the street." I said, "Repeat after me: 'If I am a bag lady on the street, I am afraid . . . .'" Fiona said, "Of being hungry and alone." I said, "If I am hungry and alone, I am afraid . . . ." Fiona said, "Of suffering." I said, "If I am suffering, I am afraid . . . ." Fiona said, "I will die."

At the core of everyone's fears is the fear that "I will die." In one sense, it may be true; moving forward in your life may require the death of a story or an identity or set of stories that you have come to identify with as who you think you are. But like the caterpillar that entered the cocoon believing it was going to die, it emerged in the end as the butterfly. The truth is that our old stories often must die for us to become who we really are.

The Illusion of Fear

There are two types of fear. The first is psychological—there is no immediate threat of danger—it is only the perception of what is happening that is creating fear (anxiety). The second is environmental, in which there is an actual threat of danger present such as a person pointing a gun at you. The first type of fear is the most common form of fear and billions of dollars a year are spent on pharmaceutical medications to quell psychological fear and anxiety.

When a fear is perceived, whether environmental or psychological, the body responds by going into the "fight or flight" response. This response can be characterized by varying degrees of sweating and trembling, as well as chest pain, shortness of breath, fidgeting, feeling like you're going to die or go crazy, hot flushes or cold chills, rapid and shallow breathing, tensed muscles, nausea, dizziness, or rapid heart-beat. While environmental fear serves to alert us to real imminent threat and danger and is typically temporary, people suffering from psychological fear are living in fear *constantly*—a fear that's not real and where no imminent danger is present. People are terribly afraid to feel because of the stories they are telling themselves about what might happen when they do. But what so many do not understand about fear is that fear can be a powerful pathway and ally to realizing the truth of our divine nature and the limitlessness of our potential. Fear can actually encourage your abilities to succeed.

> *Exposing ourselves to our personal demons is the best way to move past them.*
>
> Psychology Today

Freedom from Fear

As my skydiving partner began counting, time slowed down. I recall it like one of those slow-motion scenes from the movie *The Matrix*. As I looked out into the vast space of nothingness in front of me, in a state of total awareness, I felt something deep and intense rise from within my belly. The feeling felt strikingly similar to witnessing the moment when a sick loved one knows that it's their time to go. In that poignant and powerful moment, just seconds before I knew I was about to jump into the unknown, I was both filled with an overwhelming sadness and a tremendous sense of gratitude as I realized that the moment I jumped, I would be leaving a part of myself behind on the plane. I was leaving behind the part of myself who had been so scared to live her truth but who had done her best to protect me in the only way she knew how—by hiding me from life. She had only wanted for me to be safe. She had been my emotional body-guard, but through her intentions to constantly protect me, she had also limited my capacity to live my life to its fullest.

I spoke a silent thank you to that fearful part of myself I would be leaving behind on the plane. In my heart I spoke the words: *Thank you. I forgive you. I love you for protecting me and now it's time for me to let you go.* As the tears welled up inside my eyes, I saw an image in my mind of that old version of myself walk out of the darkness and into the light, and I felt my heart and soul open and expand. I could see that the old version of myself was not free. I suddenly knew in that precise moment that everything happens for a reason. I was *exactly* where I was supposed to be in my life, and everything was unfolding perfectly. I had the faith and the belief that everything would be okay, and then I leaped from the plane into the light.

As I flew like I a bird, racing toward the ground, I felt totally and utterly free. As I looked out and saw the earth below, tears began streaming down my cheeks. Never before had I seen anything so beautiful. Life in all its glory.

I felt a smile erupt on my wind-blown face, and I yelled to the clouds with an abundant joy: "Thank you for my amazing life!"

When love, light and truth are present, darkness and fear will scatter.

Kate's Story

I worked with a client many years ago who, at the time, was married and had two teenage children. She was approximately 45 pounds overweight at the time we met and her whole life was governed by her fears. Fear of social environments. Fear of saying what was on her mind. Fear of confrontation. Fear of her feelings, etc. One of her major fears was of *being alone.* Her husband would often travel for work and while, on one hand, she enjoyed the free time her husband's absence gave her, on the other hand, she felt an unfamiliar feeling of aloneness arise. Her feeling of aloneness was especially powerful at night when the kids were in bed, the lights were off, and she was left with her own thoughts in the dark.

When Kate was not distracted by her life and had nothing to do, her mind began its chattering, and her attention was attracted to the stories in her head which she also believed. I asked her, "What scares you about being alone?" She replied, "I feel as though I don't exist—it's like I'm not alive." When I asked Kate what she did with this fear, she said, "I go down to my kitchen and eat."

When we dug deeper into this fear, as I'm inviting you to do, Kate realized, as I did, and all my other clients eventually do, that when we enter into and go beyond our fears, not only do we *not* die—we become the butterfly. We rise to the truth of who we really want to be—the truth of who we are on the inside. We experience clarity.

Courage is not the lack of fear, but the ability to face it.
John B. Putnam Jr.

It's important at this juncture to recognize that our presenting fears (the ones we are aware of right now) are usually *not* the root cause fear that prevents us from transforming. These are just the ones our ego-mind tells about us as a means to distract us from having to recognize the truth—so that the fear itself can remain alive. The more attention we give to our *presenting* fears, such as going around and around in our head with all the stories that support these fears and cause us to experience anxiety, the more we divert our attention away from the real fear that is buried deep inside, and is the one we need to expose and face to set ourselves free.

Here are some of the presenting fears I have witnessed in clients over the past decade. None of which, when I dug a little deeper, were what was actually holding my client back from being who they wanted to be, living the life they wanted and having the body they wanted to occupy. See if you can identify with any of these, and then ask yourself the question: *What am I afraid of?*

- Afraid of exercises requiring balance
- Afraid of falling
- Afraid of exercises that require being on the floor—not be able to get up
- Afraid of appearing foolish

- Afraid to be by themselves
- Afraid to sit still for more than 10 seconds
- Afraid to investigate the space and silence between their thoughts
- Afraid to say "no"
- Afraid to exercise boundaries
- Afraid to express anger, sadness, or their true feelings
- Afraid to honestly tell loved ones how they feel
- Afraid to try new foods or embark on a new eating regimen
- Afraid to give up sugar
- Afraid to tell the truth
- Afraid of running out of breath
- Afraid of injuring themselves
- Afraid to exercise in public
- Afraid of being vulnerable and out of control
- Afraid of passing gas during exercise (flatulence during exercise is very common, by the way, and nothing to be embarrassed about)
- Afraid to try on clothes in clothing stores
- Afraid to travel in an airplane
- Afraid to ask questions of their doctor
- Afraid to go within their bodies
- Afraid to end their addictions
- Afraid to answer the question: "What are you *feeling* in your body right now?"
- And many more . . .

Transforming Fear

The only way to transform a fear is to acknowledge it, embrace it, and walk right into the center of it through our awareness and our actions. When we act despite our fears, we are embracing our fears and powerfully going beyond them in order to get more information—information that will set us free. That's how we can use our fears to propel us forward in life in the direction of where we want to go. This is what my client Patricia experienced when she walked into the center of her fears during one of our sessions.

Her presenting issue, aside from her weight, was that she was unhappy in her marriage.

By facing our fears we can exit our self-imposed prisons and become who we want to be.

Patricia's Story

When Patricia and I met, she was carrying more than 260 pounds on her small frame and was unhappy in her marriage, which she felt impaired her ability to grow. A mother of three young children, Patricia is a confident, capable, charismatic, and empathic woman whose awareness of the needs of others is paramount in everything she does. In fact, she felt that the needs of others were more important than her own. So I asked Patricia the same question I asked Fiona and Kate: "What are you afraid of?"

On first inquiry, Patricia couldn't answer this question (which is common, as the mind can actively block our ability to perceive the answer), so I invited her to enter into a state of relaxation and then I asked her to be *aware* of the question and simply notice what sensations, memories, thoughts, or stories arose within her awareness. She did as I invited and then said, "I can recall a time when I was eight. I was abused, and my parents did not believe me." I acknowledged her courage and then invited her to see herself inside her mind at the young and tender age of eight. I asked her what this younger version of herself had needed at that time that she didn't receive, the receiving of which would allow her fears to dissolve. She said, "I needed to feel loved and protected." I invited her to imagine that her younger self was easily able to receive this love and protection, and she said she couldn't, which is common. She was struggling to give her younger self the love she wanted her to receive because she herself did not feel worthy of such love—giving it to herself felt very difficult. So I shifted my direction with Patricia and I asked her to focus on her younger self once more, to see her younger self suffering and in desperate need of something to ease her pain. When she told me she could picture herself clearly, I said, "Now imagine yourself as a little girl and imagine she is *your daughter.*" In an instant, Patricia was in tears. The thought of her daughter in as much pain as she'd experienced was immediately overwhelming. As she visualized this image inside her mind, she said, "I love you, it was not your fault," and then she said to me, "I want to hug her and hold her." I said, "Then hug and hold her with all the love that you have, and as you do, picture that little girl now *as you.*"

Empowering Information

While this process of healing took place within Patricia, some new information about herself got revealed. Patricia realized that this event was the beginning of her emotional addiction to food. When she told her parents what had happened, they then shipped her off to be with her aunt, where she stayed for several weeks. When she returned home, her mother said she had almost doubled in size. With nobody to talk to and share her feelings with, she stuffed them deep inside herself, along with who she really was, and turned to the comfort of food. It then became a behavior she would use to suppress all her feelings until we began working together. You cannot stuff down your feelings and expect to arise in your truth. Part of our truth *is* our feelings, and when we suppress them into our physical bodies, we suppress ourselves. Eventually the body will begin pushing back. What does it feel like when this happens? It feels like *fear* and anxiety.

Forgiveness

Patricia also needed to forgive her parents, which she did with exceptional grace and humility. She became aware, as we all eventually do, that her parents had done the best they could based on the levels of awareness and the inner resources they had at the time. Patricia was also able to recognize that she herself had made many mistakes with her own children, as we all do, and that not once had she ever stopped loving her children. This helped her realize that her parents had never stopped loving her. They had simply done what they'd modelled from *their* parents who in turn had done the same—

modeling and learning the same pathology from *their* parents. But once we break the pattern in ourselves, we cease the continuation of that pathology in our children.

Our greatest fear is not that are we inadequate, but that we are powerful beyond measure. It is our light, not our darkness, that frightens us most.
Marianne Williamson

The next step in Patricia's healing process was to bring awareness to how her fear had manifested inside her relationship with her husband and how she had been afraid to step into her true magnificence and live her beautiful truth.

Patricia's biggest complaint in being married to her husband was that she did not feel free to be herself. Yet as I guided Patricia to inquire more deeply into this idea and story, she awoke to the truth that her husband was not the reason for her stunted growth, but that she was the one responsible. She came to realize that she had *chosen* her husband—nobody had forced her—because he was the perfect enabler, allowing Patricia to remain in her fears and limiting stories. She could use her husband as an excuse.

When Patricia did not get the love and safety she had wanted from her parents, she decided in that moment that who she was, the truth of her nature, was not good enough or worthy enough to be loved. So she buried that self, and took on another identity (one whose focus was on everyone else) to cope. This identity limited her life but at least she didn't have to *feel* her emotional pain. Then she did what many people with food addictions have done—she turned to food for comfort and safety. But because our truth doesn't want to be buried—it was not supposed to be the lamp we put under the bed, but rather a light to shine and brighten our world—it perseveres in trying to get our attention. It says, "Notice me, see me, hear me, free me—let me shine my light, please!" And we say, "Shut up!" and then go order a pizza.

The Truth Will Set You Free

Patricia's husband was not the problem, though it was true his behaviors were not supportive. However, Patricia's power lay not in changing her husband, but in being 100 percent responsible for her own behaviors. What this responsibility looks like is *being in our truth*—in other words, taking responsibility for and honoring our feelings by expressing them and giving them our attention.

Patricia needed to move beyond her fears, not by hiding behind them or resisting them, but by bravely walking into them. Patricia needed to start telling the truth about her deepest feelings and become transparently honest with the people around her, especially her husband. She needed to start living the life that was etched in her heart, and that's exactly what she did. She also dropped weight, by the way.

Denial

Denial (de-Nile) may well be a river in Egypt, but it's also a major obstacle to transformation.

One of the biggest tricks our minds can use to divert our attention away from our true fears is through the act of denial.

Several years ago I trained and counseled a wonderful woman who was so scared of addressing the fears lodged in her emotional body that she had mastered the art of denial. More than 200 pounds overweight, this woman flat out told me at our initial session together that her goal was only to improve her health—she did not need to lose any weight. Perhaps she could afford to drop a few pounds here and there, but she wanted me to know that she was totally comfortable with her body and that it's what you think about your body that matters, not what your body actually looks like. On one hand, this sounded like a healthy statement of self-love and self-acceptance. But I also knew that it wasn't the whole truth, as I knew she couldn't really be "totally comfortable" with being obese.

This same woman would also come to our training sessions armed with a library full of stories and goals and intentions she would never meet. She constantly compared her body to the body of others, and it was almost impossible to stop her from talking. As soon as I invited her to be present to her body while performing any exercise and just simply focus on her breathing—she would either ask an irrelevant question or comment that something about the exercise was difficult. She was doing this to avoid being present to the moment, and present to her physical body, which houses her emotional self.

When I gently suggested it was possible she was not happy with her body and possibly even her life, and that it appeared to me that she was living in denial, she snapped at me like a wild dog and said, "I have no idea what you mean!"

One day she decided on a goal (one of many) to lose "just a few pounds" so she could wear a strapless dress to a friend's wedding. But when the wedding rolled around and she wore a suit instead, I inquired about what had happened. She told me that even though her goal had been to wear a strapless dress, she'd decided at the last minute to be unique and different because she didn't want to be like everyone else. She also said that she had decided to wear a suit with a sleeveless top underneath, which was "pretty much the same as a strapless dress." Clearly it was not!

Denial is a powerful energy that is really just another way to self-preserve and protect what wants to remain hidden within. This client would tell me repeatedly during our sessions together about what a wonderful and delightful relationship she had with her children and her husband. On observation of her relationship with one of her sons, and after listening to her stories about her communications and relationship with her husband, it was apparent to me that these relationships were clearly dysfunctional and unhealthy. There was not a lot of truth and transparency in her family. She would often refer to her son as her BFF (best friend forever) and, even though he was also obese, would repeatedly tell me what a great body he had, and how she wished his disillusioned classmates at school would stop calling him "fat."

She would avoid at all costs having to use emotional words to describe how she was feeling and would instead give me a lengthy description of what she thought, which on the surface appeared positive and empowering. Problem was, it was a total lie. Inside she was a cacophony of rage, resentment, guilt, shame, and grief, all of which was sitting on a bed of overwhelming sadness masking itself as fear.

It took me more than two years to get this client to see the truth about how truly unhappy she was as a parent, in her marriage and in her life in general, and how she'd become someone else to please those around her, who she felt didn't love her as she truly was. But how could anyone love the truth of who she was when she was constantly showing up as someone else? It was only when she recognized her denial that her journey of healing and transformation began.

Worthiness

No matter how a fear initially shows up, in *every* single client I've worked with, the root fear that fuels all their fears is the belief that who they are is not good enough. They believe they're not deserving of unconditional love. For every single client I've worked with, this belief stemmed from an experience or event early in childhood when they felt rejected by someone whose love they desperately needed at that time—namely their mom or dad or some significant other. So to avoid having to ever suffer from this rejection again, they suppressed their true self and adopted a different identity that protected them from ever having to feel this emotional pain again.

At the core of every amazing and magnificent human being is the idea that who they are is not good enough—not worthy of unconditional love. But when we realize that this belief is simply an idea that was innocently accepted as truth at some early point in our childhood, without our say in the matter, we can then realize that the only love we ever really need to transform is our own. Self-loving is not about being egotistical or bathing in a pool of shallow showy arrogance. Self-love is about loving the essence of who you are, and letting the truth of that essence shine through you. Then we can receive the love that's all around us.

We don't necessarily have to love all our behaviors, every part of our body, or even, let's say, our hair, if it's the sort of hair we wished we didn't have. Self-love is about having a deep and profound respect and appreciation for the divinity of the beauty and love that runs through you, which is the real truth of who you are. The more you can come to love and respect the essence of your being, the more you can start to appreciate all the parts you previously didn't like about yourself, such as your hair or your hips—the very hips you may have once thought were too wide. You can start to see the greater magnificence that's housed within us all, and understand that "beauty" reaches far beyond the physical body. When this love for self begins taking place, you will cease wanting to harm and abuse your body through excess eating or the refusal to exercise, because you will treasure and value the physical form that houses your magnificent self.

Beyond Fear

At this point in your journey, the obstacle that now stands between the body and the life you want is likely fear. What prevents you from being present to your emotional body while reaching for another cookie is fear. Yet fear is not what stunts our transformation; it's our resistance to its presence that causes harm. Fear is not something you need to be afraid of. It's just information wanting to enter your awareness to help you know yourself better.

The goal should not be to run from your fears, but to confront, embrace, and transform them into fuel that we can use to become who we want to be.

Learning from Our Fear

When we can learn to see fear and its forms of emotional disguise, such as anger, anxiety, guilt, depression, and shame simply as pertinent "information" arising from within the body and ego-mind to teach us something, we can calmly and clearly assess the source of its origins and find out what it needs us to know. The more we understand about our fears, the less power they have to cause us to panic and control us. The more we realize why they are there, the greater our potential to transform.

THOUGHT PROVOKER

• *What are you afraid of?*

Going Within

When I invite my clients to go within themselves, almost immediately they become fearful because of all the stories their mind is telling them, such as: *It's not safe to look inside, and something bad is going to happen here.* So many of us have been hardwired with the belief that who we really are is not good enough, and it is therefore dangerous to be honest about our inner truth.

When I faced my fears by jumping from that plane, I let the truth of my fears be known to myself. I realized through my fears that it was my deeply held belief of my own unworthiness that was holding me back in my life. Once I realized that who I am is loved simply for just being me, I lost my need to seek out love and approval from others and I was free to just, well, be me.

Now that I understand that I am always safe in the eternal arms of the thread of love that flows through everything in life, my fears no longer disarm me or cause me to panic. Instead they fuel my desires and intentions in life and make me more aware of myself and what I am here to learn.

Fear of Insanity

We are all terrified of losing our mental faculties, of being vulnerable and helpless in the face of hurt and rejection. Many are afraid they will go insane if they allow their feelings to surface and if they truly face their fears. But in all my years both personally and professionally, I have never once witnessed a client go mad or die from facing their fears. However, what I have seen, time and time again, is the lifting and shedding of years of emotional burden, heartache, and darkness. I have seen, over and over again, this fear and pain transformed into the light of self-love and acceptance. I have seen tears of joy, relief, and gratitude, as people bathe in the ocean of their newfound freedom—fearless to be the truth of who they are.

Are you ready to face the truth of what is holding you back so you can be free to live the life you desire?

When you walk through the valley of fear, it's a bit like driving into fog. You feel uneasy at first because you can't see beyond the fog, but you persevere because you know that the only way to get to the other side is to drive through it. So with faith and trust as your only guides, you continue forward, because you know that where you've come from served its purpose, but it no longer serves where you are going. Eventually the fog begins to disperse, and you find yourself on the other side—in the clarity of the light. In the heavenly arms of love and grace.

Are you ready to let go of that which no longer serves you?

Are you ready to exit your fearful chrysalis and let your butterfly emerge?

Practices: Beyond Fear

The following practices are designed to help you gain a better understanding about your fears. Since your fears are the only barrier to your transformation right now, it is important to embrace this exercise with a deep and heartfelt intention to finally release that which you know no longer serves you. If I were with you at this moment, I would hold your hand, look you in the eyes and remind you that you are safe. But since I am not with you in person, I can only hope that the words on this page are enough. I promise you that you will not die. It's very possible you will experience some emotions though, but by now you've realized your emotions are nothing to be afraid of. They are the gateway to your transformation—which, may I gently remind you, is what you want and is why you're ready for this book. You are safe. You are loved. All is well. It's time now to release your fears.

To best prepare for this practice, I invite you to find somewhere quiet where you will not be interrupted for the duration. I invite you to bring with you to this practice anything that evokes a feeling of safety within you, such as an object of some sort (it could be a book, a stone, the Bible, a photograph of someone who evokes feelings of love and safety within you), and begin with the centering meditation from the Introduction. The following practice is a two-part exercise. Please do them back-to-back if you can.

Part One: Become Aware of Your Fears

1. In your journal or in the journal pages in the back of this book, write down all your fears you are aware of.

2. Read through your list and recognize that each of these fears is showing up as a symptom of a much deeper fear.

3. Investigate each fear by using the phrase below, digging deeper each time until you can go no further. (Refer back to Fiona's story if you need to remind yourself how to do this exercise.) "If I am_____, I am afraid of_____."

Part Two: Transforming Your Fears

1. Access a loving state of awareness.

2. Hold in your mind the deepest fear you are aware of.

3. Observe where you feel this fear *most* is in your body.

4. If it had a color, shape, and texture, what color, shape, and texture would it be?

5. Imagine your fear as a little frightened child and ask the fear, "What is your story? Why are you so afraid?" (Notice if any memories arise within your awareness and trust that they are there for a reason and hold a special message and learning for you.)

6. Ask the fear when it originated (again, notice if anything arises—see step 5).

7. Inquire about the stories attached to the fear and notice any limiting beliefs.

8. Assume there is a lesson to be had from this fear, and ask the fear what it wants you to know as it relates to your challenges with your body and your desire to transform.

9. Ask the fear what it needs to *believe* and *feel* to be free to leave your body. (Notice what arises.)

10. Journal and capture all the lessons and thank your fear for sharing.

11. Finally, meditate on your fear in a state of awareness with the intention to take a new action that will permanently erase that fear as an issue in your life. Then when you're ready, take new action.

CHAPTER 9

ACTION: TURNING DREAMS INTO REALITY

Action is the foundational key to all success.
Pablo Picasso

Knowing is not enough. We must apply. Willing is not enough. We must do.
Bruce Lee

O ne of the most difficult questions for many of my clients to answer is the question: *What do you want?* What do you want to experience in your life, and what changes do you want to see in your body and why? When clients begin their transformation journey with me, we always begin with a "Setting Goals and Intentions Session." I want to know what my clients want as their outcome, as it helps me plan and prepare our time together, it gives me insight into their deeper dreams and desires, and it gives my clients a pathway to follow and ignites their motivation. Without knowing the answer to the question, What do I want?, it is impossible to know what actionable steps need to be taken to achieve desired results.

What do you want to change in your life and body and why?

Desire Precedes Motivation

To take the action necessary to transform both your body and your life, you need to awaken the state of *desire* within you. Without desire you cannot sustain unstoppable drive and motivation, which you are going to need if you want to succeed. Without drive and motivation, the action steps you need to take will not get taken and nothing will ever change for you. Everything will remain the same for you—and considering how far you've already come through this book, I know this isn't what you want.

So before you embark on the action portion of your physical transformation, begin with establishing your *goals and intentions*. In other words, know in advance *exactly* what you want with as much specificity and detail as possible. For instance, do you want to be able to feel comfortable in your clothes and shop for clothes in regular stores, not plus-size stores? Do you want walk with confidence in a bikini on the beaches of Acapulco with your head held high? Do you want to lose a specific number of inches from your waist so you reduce your health risk and are able to wear that fabulous pair of jeans you bought several years ago? Do you want to get off your blood pressure or cholesterol medication and shrink your heart chambers? Do you want to be able to run around the block with your children and not gasp for breath? Do you want to be able to carry your groceries easily and effortlessly from the grocery store to your car without wincing in pain? Do you want to run your first-ever 5K race and complete it in 25 minutes? Do you want to become a yoga instructor, set up your own studio, and inspire others to love and take care of their bodies, too? Do you want to make love to your partner with the lights on? Do you want to be able to cross your legs comfortably and no longer experience chafing or rashes between your thighs? Do you want to get up and down from the floor easily and effortlessly without feeling clumsy and embarrassed or that you might fall and hurt yourself? Do you want to sit comfortably in the seats at the cinema or in an airplane and not feel suffocated by the seatbelt or feeling as though you're encroaching on the space of the person beside you? Do you want to have control and power over what you put in your mouth? And also, *why* do you want these things?

If you have built castles in the air, your work need not be lost; that is where they should be. Now put the foundation under them.

Henry David Thoreau

Practice: Goals and Intentions

In this chapter, you're not going to wait until the end to do the practices. I want to encourage you to take action now! Here you're going to set your goals and intentions.

1. In your journal answer the question "What do you want?" with as much detail as possible. These are your goals and intentions.

2. When you have listed your goals and intentions, re-read your list and notice if you have used positive and transformational language, or limiting language. For example, "I no longer want to be fat and feel ugly" is an example of a goal and intention that is written in a disempowering way and with limiting language. When you read this statement, your mind will focus exclusively on "fat" and "ugly." These are not what I consider empowering or transformational words, because when you read the words "fat" and "ugly," your emotions respond accordingly and put you in a disempowered rather than an empowered state of mind and feeling. Instead, you want to write what you want *exactly* as you want it. Instead of "I no longer want to be fat and feel ugly," you could write, "I want to feel comfortable and confident in my body, and when I look

in the mirror, I love what I see and I feel beautiful." Can you see how the last sentence evokes different emotional responses? Our emotions drive our actions, and if we feel ugly and fat, we'll be more inclined to keep eating than to start exercising because we won't feel good about ourselves. But if we are responding emotionally to the words "beautiful, comfortable, and confident," we feel positive and motivated to move our bodies and take good care of them. Remember to also ask yourself the question, *why* do I want these things? The answer to this question will awaken a deeper understanding within you more closely linked with your deepest values in life and what will motivate you more to do the action steps needed to achieve your goals. If our goals don't align with our values, we simply won't be motivated to make any new changes.

3. Once you've ensured all your goals and intentions are written in empowering and transformational language, I'd like you to put an end date beside each one. For instance, "It is August 1, 2015, and I am able to cross my legs comfortably and easily. I feel confident in my own skin, and when I'm feeling confident, I can powerfully show up in the world as my true me." An end date helps us plan and prepare. If we know where the finish line is, we can plan and strategize accordingly. By adding in the end date you can also write your goals in the present tense. For instance, "It is August 1, 2015, and I am able to cross my legs comfortably and easily." As opposed to, "It is August 1, 2015, and I will be able to cross my legs comfortably and easily." Notice the change in feeling when you state in the present tense as opposed to the future.

4. Once you have all your goals and intentions dated and written in transformational language with as much detail as possible, your next step is to decide what action steps and resources are necessary to achieve each goal and intention. You might need to hire a personal trainer. You might need to clear out your kitchen cupboards of all sugary and unhealthy foods and write out a new grocery list that's jam-packed with nutrient-dense, fat-burning vegetables, lean meats, and fruits. Maybe you need to create a schedule to accommodate a daily workout. Maybe you need to have a conversation with your family to let them know about your

expectations and what kind of support you'd like from them. Whatever resources you need and whatever steps need to be taken to achieve each of your goals, write them down.

5. Finally, I want you to create a "My Awesome Life" Inspiration Board. This involves buying a large big piece of poster board and spending one to two hours gluing onto the board images, words, colors, and symbols (these images can come from anywhere—i.e., magazines, the Internet, your personal papers, or a photo collection) that best represent the life and body you want to have. In the center of the board write the words "My Awesome Life," and then grab colored pens, scissors, paints, a pile of magazines to clip out desired words and phrases, and a glue stick, and begin. On my board, I have written, painted, or glued down words like *love, health, oneness, fitness, God, gratitude,* and *making a difference,* as well as positive quotes, scriptures, meaningful mantras, lines from different poets, heart symbols, photographs of nature scenes, pictures of people exercising, and animals—all the things I want to experience and have show up in my life. When I competed for the first time as a fitness athlete, which I did to inspire and motivate others to see what's possible when we put our minds to something, I created a specific board just for this event. I had set the intention to place and take home a trophy, so my board was filled with images of other fitness athletes holding trophies. I also put a photograph of myself on the board with the words "First Place Winner!" written underneath. I didn't win my first competition, but I came in third—twice—and my board helped me to achieve this outcome. It also helped me to stay centered and focused and helped me to plan, prepare, and stay on track. It kept me motivated and excited, and the words and images inspired me every day to keeping going and to never give up. Every day I sat in front of my board and *visualized* and *imagined* that everything on my board was happening in that very moment in my life. I would always end these sessions expressing my deepest gratitude—giving thanks for the many blessings I already have in my life and praying for the courage, guidance and mental and emotional strength to succeed, and for my

achievements to be of benefit and inspiration to others. I invite you and encourage you to do the same.

If you find for any reason that you're not able to *know* exactly what you want, this is an indication that you may still be emotionally blocked and living in fear. If this is the case, I encourage you to revisit chapters 5 and 8. I also encourage you to engage in the following Heart's Desire practice (which is useful even if you know what you want, as it will invite you to go a little deeper).

Practice: Heart's Desire

1. Go into the Centering Meditation (see Introduction).
2. Draw your attention to your heart center. Imagine your heart opening up so that you may have a conversation with it about its deepest desires and wishes for you.
3. Ask yourself this question: *If I did not care what other people thought, if money was no object, and if I had a magic wand, what would I do and be in my life?*
4. Write down your answers in your journal.
5. While still focusing on your heart center, make a list of what's important to you in your life.
6. Circle the top five values on your list.
7. Ask your heart center the following questions: "Am I really living these values? If not, why not? What am I afraid of?" (Observe and acknowledge any fears, and then process these fears using the practices at the end of chapter 8.)
8. Do an internal integrity and honesty check. Are you being totally honest with yourself about what you want and about what's important to you? Or are you holding back for some reason? Do you fear rejection or judgment from others? Do you fear something else? What are you afraid of? (Again, I invite you to observe and acknowledge any fears, and then process these fears using the practices at the end of chapter 8.)

9. Then ask your heart this question: *If you had only one wish for me in my life, and you wanted me to experience this wish because you love me, what would this wish be?*

10. Capture all your responses and insights in your journal.

Visualization

Before I do anything, I first see it with crystal clarity in my mind and I feel it in my body. Once I can feel it and I've seen it made manifest in my mind, I know with certainty I can create it.

The soul never thinks without a picture.

Aristotle

Visualization and prayer is a simple, yet powerful, technique that throws more fuel on the fire of your passion. While you stay focused on your daily action steps, you can also engage your imagination to achieve your goals and desires even faster. When you take the time to regularly visualize the life you want, you generate the energy and inspiration you need to take positive action. By seeing yourself completing each step and each goal first within your mind's eye, you actually increase the potential of your dream life becoming your reality. Your positive imagination not only fuels your motivation, it activates the Law of Attraction to bring to you all the opportunities and people you need to accomplish your ultimate goals.

There is a difference between fantasizing or wishful thinking and creatively visualizing your intentions and goals. Fantasizing and wishful thinking are generally motivated by negative impulses. For instance, if you are wishing you looked like a Victoria Secret model while you are feeling tired, angry, and fat, you are not creating that possibility for yourself; you are only reinforcing what you don't want, which is to feel tired, angry, and fat. Effective visualization can only happen when you have accepted yourself and your circumstances as they are in the present.

I know accepting yourself as you are may sound difficult, as it is your dissatisfaction with yourself and your current situation that is driving you to want something better out of life, but you cannot move forward in your life without first affirming and appreciating yourself as you are. Your dissatisfaction and discomfort serve only as a wakeup call, a reminder that you are worthy of the best body and life you can imagine for yourself. You must pay attention to this wakeup call without using it as a way to further abuse yourself.

If you were to lovingly see yourself as your own child, you might be able to feel the compassion for yourself that you must cultivate in order to begin to create the changes you want. Once you have found a way to feel a little bit more self-accepting, learning to direct your visualizations will be easy! After all, visualizing is something that comes completely naturally and easily. What I will do here is talk about how to super-charge your visualizations so that they truly support your heart-felt desires and goals. You can create anything you want if you think it, feel it, value it, and believe it to be true! As you move forward in this process, you may become aware of beliefs you hold that are preventing you from fully visualizing, and manifesting what you want. If you find this to be the case, I suggest you review chapter 2.

Visualization is a powerful, creative technique that works for scientific, psychological, emotional, and spiritual reasons. When you focus on something specific over a period of time, there is a neurological connection made in your brain—a groove or pathway is formed—which helps you keep that focus. This is how habits are formed and why it is often challenging to change old habits and create new ones. Visualization works similarly to hypnosis in that your subconscious mind is reprogrammed to adopt new beliefs and attitudes, ones that overtly support rather than unconsciously sabotage your desires and dreams.

The positive image you are visualizing of the life and body you want makes you feel better, and as you feel better, you become more enthusiastic and motivated to take the action steps that will help you realize your dreams. By engaging in the practice of visualizing greater possibilities for yourself, you open up to inspiration (which is defined by *Merriam-Webster* as "a divine influence or action on a person believed to qualify him or her to receive and communicate sacred revelation"). By using the simple tool of visualization for personal transformation, you are giving yourself the opportunity to make the changes you want with grace and ease. As you visualize, pray to God/the Universe to support you and to bring your desires into your reality.

Practice: Visualization

There are many ways to approach visualization. I will give you several different ideas and allow you to discover what works best for you.

1. Begin with the Centering Meditation (see Introduction).
2. One of the most effective ways to make sure you have a happy and productive day, especially if you are busy and have very specific goals, is to visualize yourself going through your day step by step. See yourself waking up with energy, enthusiastically working out, happily eating a healthy, delicious breakfast, joyfully going to work, eating a healthy lunch with friends, getting your work done easily, having pleasant encounters with colleagues, receiving compliments, getting home effortlessly in spite of traffic, fixing a good, nutritious dinner, enjoying family meal time, and having a fun, sexy, or relaxing evening with your partner. See yourself falling asleep easily and sleeping so deeply so that you feel replenished the next morning. This is something you can do before you go to sleep at night and just before you get up in the morning.
3. Visualizing your more far-reaching goals can be done simultaneously or at a different time of day. It is important to find a time when you have a few moments of peace and quiet to focus your thoughts on the pictures you want. When you sit down to visualize, close your eyes and take a few deep, cleansing breaths. Consciously relax your body, and place your hands over your heart to center your attention there. When you feel calm, conjure the image you want of yourself, not only how you would like to look, but how you would

like to feel. In my experience, it is sometimes more empowering and effective to focus on how you would like to feel in your life rather than how you would like to look or what you would like to have. I also like to pray and give thanks for turning my dreams and desires into reality.

4. There is nothing wrong with wanting to be a size 6 or 120 pounds or wanting to have a Mercedes or your own private jet for that matter, but when it comes to visualizing, if you don't achieve your material goals quickly enough, sometimes you can become discouraged and give up before you have the opportunity to create what you want. I usually recommend that you visualize a more holistic picture of yourself. In other words, see yourself in a sexy, size 6 dress at a fabulous party given in your honor, surrounded by your loving family and friends. See, hear, and feel their compliments. You can even visualize the smell and taste of your intentions. Tune into your energy; see and feel how elated and energized you are. Not only are you leaner and beautiful, you are happy and glowing, filled with energy and confidence. You love yourself and you love your life.

5. Find images of yourself and your life that you can connect to over and over again. Persistence pays off and the more frequently you can energize the image of yourself and your life that you want to create, the more likely it is to materialize. I also encourage you to remember that this is a creative exercise and if you feel inspired to shift your routine, alter your images and/or take a specific action in service to realizing your dreams, do it! By honoring your desires and meditating on your dreams, you expand your consciousness and open yourself to guidance from God. You will know you are being truly guided when you feel uplifted, elated, excited, inspired, energized, or emotionally moved.

6. It is important to stay positive. This is not an opportunity to list your dislikes or to compare yourself unfavorably to someone else. This is about seeing your highest potential and energizing it by dreaming on it!

Only put off until tomorrow what you are willing to die having left undone.

Pablo Picasso

Setting Action Steps

At the end of the day, the only way you are going to see any physical transformation in your body and desired changes in your life is through consistent and intentional action. Only you are capable of your turning your dreams into reality and taking action is how you will make this happen. Your dreams and desires will remain pictures inside your mind until you take action toward making them a reality in your life. The difference between those who succeed in reaching their goals and those who don't comes down to one necessary behavior—*action.* You must act, and you must keep acting until you achieve what you want. You must not accept mediocrity or stop acting because times get tough. That would be like pulling out of a race because you're tired when the finish line is just ahead.

It's also important to realize that there is not really an "end goal." Once you've achieved one goal, life doesn't just suddenly stop. You will continue to create and re-invent yourself in alignment with what you want to experience next in your life. Because your values will change over time, so too, will your goals, dreams, and desires. I often tell my clients that setting goals and intentions can be like climbing a staircase. We don't climb the whole staircase in one single bound. Rather, we take one step at a time as we focus on reaching the top. We need to be present to each step and give our total attention and awareness to our journey so as not to lose our balance, and topple or fall backwards. Then when we reach the top, we experience a moment of achievement and success and hopefully a level of transformation. But it doesn't stop here. Instead, we notice another flight of stairs before us, leading upward from our path. Here we can either choose to remain on the level we have reached, or choose to embark on another journey of steps, each time recognizing that life is about the journey, not the destination. The steps represent moments in our lives—moments we will never get back and ones we don't want to rush through. Rather, we want to be present to these moments, to enjoy and experience what each step has to offer us.

There is learning, opportunity, and transformation available on every step. That's why I express gratitude so often—I am aware that each step is a gift, regardless of whether it feels easy or difficult. When you arrive at the top of your staircase, if you expect all your problems to suddenly end, or that you will not have to continue to pay attention, stay focussed or make an effort, then you will be disappointed. This is not how it is. Life is a journey of experience. It is not a race to a future moment that holds all our dreams and desires and thus completes our life. No. This is the purpose of each step. You can experience your dreams and desires on each step. You can have everything you want on each step. You can even have everything you want right now, so long as you're willing to change your attitude. The purpose of this chapter is not to push you to get to a final destination where your health and life are concerned. The purpose of this chapter is to help you develop a lifestyle and way of being that will give you the opportunity to make each moment of your life's journey fulfilling—a journey that opens you to the desires of your heart and allows your soul to truly strive and evolve so that you may experience the magnificence that is you.

All that's required is to take one step. One step at a time.

Rome was not built in a day, and when we put together a puzzle, we do so one piece at a time. What's going to be the first action step for you? What is the first piece of your life's puzzle?

Any action is better than no action at all.
Norman Vincent Peale

Here is an example of a set of action steps to bring further clarity to the process of defining the action steps needed to achieve your goals and intentions.

Sample Goal and Intention: By May 2, 2014, I will be off my high-blood pressure medication and wearing my favorite pair of jeans, because that means I am honoring my body and living my truth.

Action Steps for Above Goal and Intention:

1. Hang my favorite pair of jeans on the wall in my bedroom.
2. Hire a personal trainer to help me improve my strength and fitness and lose weight.
3. Speak to my doctor about what I need to do to begin weaning myself off my medication.
4. Set up a blog online and begin blogging my journey for accountability and to inspire others.
5. Eat five healthy meals a day that consist of fresh vegetables, fruit, and lean meats.
6. Record my daily progress in my journal.
7. Express gratitude and pray/meditate every morning for five minutes.
8. Buy a new pair of running shoes.
9. Ask Suzie if she'd be interested in going on morning walks with me.
10. Meditate daily on my 'My Awesome Life' Board.

Action is always your next move.
Napoleon Hill

Dreams become reality when intentions become action.
Unknown

Planning and Scheduling

You have to have a plan if you're going to succeed. Getting up each day and hoping life will just give you what you want is like expecting a goldfish to suddenly leap out of its bowl and start riding a bicycle. Life is a collaborative process. It will give you what you want—everything in fact—but action is required on your part. Action, faith, and the unwavering belief that you are loved beyond measure and capable of living the life etched in your heart.

It is important that you begin every single day knowing your intentions. If you don't know your intentions, you won't know what action to take and when. Sometimes what you intend won't always happen exactly as you expect, but believe me, it is always for a very good reason. Sometimes what *we* want is modified for the purpose of supporting the grander whole, of which we are an integral part, and which is intimately connected to us. What we do affects the whole. Our actions and intentions *mean* something. Life gives back what we put out. Your one positive intention and action helps to add joy, love, inspiration, possibility, hope, and happiness to the whole. The outcome of your goals and intentions doesn't only affect you in a positive way—it affects everyone.

It is also important that you keep your mind on track and that your thoughts remain positive and empowering. Begin each day by readjusting your mental and emotional software. Remember that what you think, believe and feel you create and experience. Each day, in every moment, be aware of your emotional body. Is it trying to get your attention? Does it need your acknowledgment and love? Make sure you are *listening* to your physical body. Does it ache? Do you feel tension, tightness, or rigidity? This is how our bodies speak to us and get our attention. The physical sensations and discomfort that arise in the body are bringing to your awareness a hidden truth that needs unveiling. At least once or more a day, check in with your physical body. Begin at your toes and work your way up to your head asking each part of your body how it feels and if it has a message for you or something it wants you to know.

Just the other day a client came in with neck pain she'd been suffering with for a week. She'd been to her chiropractor and had a massage, but the discomfort hadn't lifted. I invited her to listen to her body and invite it to share with her the reason for its discomfort. She became aware that she had been overburdening herself recently with the problems of others. She literally felt the "weight of the world on her shoulders" and had been ignoring her own needs. She left our session a little lighter and sent a text message fifteen minutes later, saying that the most remarkable thing had just happened. Her neck clicked as she was driving, and the discomfort she felt was now gone.

THOUGHT PROVOKERS

- *What is your physical body telling you right now?*
- *What are your intentions right now?*
- *What is the quality of your thoughts right now?*
- *What is occurring within your emotional body right now?*

Take One Step

Right now I invite you to put down this book and go and take just *one* action step in the direction of your goals and intentions. Maybe it's writing a loving note to yourself, registering for a class of some sort, hiring a trainer, making a healthy grocery list, saying a prayer, marking your calendar with the days you wish to work out, or setting up a blog to record your transformational journey. It doesn't matter how big or small your action step is. What matters is that you take the step. Go do it right now, and then meet me back here.

Thinking will not overcome fear, but action will.
Clement Stone

If you find any fears surfacing as you consider taking action, revisit chapter 8. In nearly all instances, our thinking *about* an action generates way more fear than the action itself.

Procrastination

So, did you take that action step, or did you find an excellent reason not to do that action step this moment? Please don't be hard on yourself. Procrastination is delaying, putting off, or deferring an action to a later time. From time to time we all find ourselves procrastinating when it would serve us better to act. The reasons why we procrastinate stem from our emotional blocks, limiting beliefs, and disempowering repetitive thoughts. At this point in the book, I hope you have uncovered many of the reasons why you have not yet taken action to improve your health and are ready now to take massive action. If, at this point, you still find yourself procrastinating, it is an indication that you are not quite ready to take action. If this is the case, I lovingly invite you to return to chapters 1 through 8, revisit all the practices and continue with these practices until you become *aware* of the reasons behind your tendency to procrastinate. You may find that you need to alter your thinking, beliefs, and emotions before you can take the action steps necessary to achieve your goals and intentions.

While writing this very chapter I found *myself* procrastinating at times—filling up my time cleaning the house, flipping through magazines and brushing the cats before I could begin writing. When I recognized *through awareness* what I was doing, and what emotional blocks and beliefs were standing in my way, I was easily able to cease my procrastinating ways and settle into writing this chapter.

Nothing will work unless you do.
Maya Angelou

The end of our inner journey is in fact the beginning of our physical journey. In Part One, we addressed our weight issues from the inside, discovering how to rise above the maze of our negative stories, beliefs, thoughts, emotions, and fears; envision our true, gorgeous, powerful selves; and create a plan to make this vision a reality.

Now it's time for the "outside" part of transforming from the inside out. No matter who you are or what your action plan may be, every*body* needs optimal fuel and movement to achieve any goal. In Part Two, you'll find easy-to-follow nutritional guidelines for fueling your body for maximum energy, as well as an equally easy-to-follow monthly workout routine to get your body fit and active so you're able to live out your beautiful truth.

PART TWO

THE PHYSICAL JOURNEY

CHAPTER 10

FUELING YOUR BODY: NUTRITION GUIDELINES

We are indeed much more than what we eat, but what we eat can nevertheless help us to be much more than what we are.
Adelle Davis

I n Part Two, you will embark on the physical part of your journey. You will be invited to follow many of the same principles and guidelines I employ and recommend to my clients to achieve your best body possible. This process of physical transformation is not about vanity, which is excessive pride in one's own abilities or attractiveness to others. It's about a truthful appreciation, gratitude, and love for our bodies that has no limits. In this chapter, we're going to begin with some practical guidelines to help you love the body you're in by giving it the fuel it needs to thrive and transform.

What Fuel Does Our Body Need?

When it comes to fueling our bodies for optimal wellness and performance, we have sadly lost touch with what our bodies need and have little sense of what is healthy. Some of us aren't even sure what real "food" is anymore. This is due to a variety of reasons: the relatively recent phenomenon of producing food for profit rather than health; the increased level of stress in our lives as a result of our technologically advanced, fast-paced, always-on-the-go lifestyles; our inability to cope emotionally with the circumstances of our lives; our lack of faith and awareness moment by moment; and our lack of attention to our body's cues that are screaming at us to pay attention to what's not working and is no longer in healthy balance. As a result, obesity has become a worldwide epidemic—people are fatter now than they have ever been—and diseases such as cancer, heart disease, adrenal fatigue, diabetes, depression, anxiety, and chronic pain disorders such as fibromyalgia are *common household names*. We are becoming sicker *and* fatter, and it can be largely attributed to what we are putting in our mouths coupled with the insane lifestyle of constant busyness so many people are now living.

To change our bodies and transform our lives, we not only need to change our relationships with our mental, emotional, spiritual, and physical selves, we also need to change our relationship with food. We need to return to the basics of healthy living: eat regular meals with healthy portions; eat clean and healthy proteins, carbohydrates, and fats; get more sleep; reduce stress; increase times of quiet and stillness; get regular exercise; spend more time in nature; and regularly practice prayer, belief, and mindfulness. We need to rediscover the true definition of the word "food" and *listen* to the way our bodies regularly communicate with us through the sensations we feel. Through knowledge, choice, faith, attention, and awareness, we can begin to consciously change what we choose to put into our mouths.

The definition of "food" is any nutritious substance that people or animals eat or drink, or that plants absorb, in order to maintain life and growth.

By engaging in discussions with various health experts, reading studies, drawing upon on my own personal and clinical experiences, and doing research about food for this book, I discovered there is a "for" and "against" argument for—well—everything. Drink milk; don't drink milk. Eat meat; don't eat meat. Eat whole grains; avoid anything with wheat. Eat brown rice; don't eat brown rice. Eat tomatoes; don't eat tomatoes. Juice your food; don't juice your food. You name it: there is a pro and con for almost everything. We also have to take into consideration personal food preferences—vegetarian or vegan, lacto-vegetarian, ovo-vegetarian, pollotarian—as well as cultural, chemical (hormonal), environmental, ethnic, and religious considerations.

That means I'm not going to give you a strict meal plan you must follow day in and day out. It would simply be irresponsible of me, and it would also rob you of your own innate ability to discover and *know* what is best for you and your body. I want to empower you with information so you can make your own choices, not simply tell you what to do. I'm going to treat you as the unique and intelligent individual that you are with unique dietary needs and invite you to consider a few nutrition general guidelines that will improve your health, enhance the quality of your life, and reshape your body—for some of you, dramatically so. These are the same guidelines I follow on a daily basis, and I implore and encourage my clients to follow these as well. This is not a diet—it's a choice and lifestyle. These guidelines have, time and time again, transformed bodies and lives for the better. You can tweak them or modify them slightly to suit your choices and preferences, but keep in mind that any major modifications or deviations outside these guidelines could delay improvement in or even negatively impact your health, wellness, and weight-loss goals. For best results, seek the guidance and expert advice of a registered holistic nutritionist or dietician.

But before I reveal these guidelines, it's important that you understand the basics about how our so-called "food" is being produced these days. Knowledge is power where your health is concerned, and it's important for you to know what is being done to your food.

Perhaps without realizing it, you are slowly being poisoned by eating food that technically isn't "food," and it is messing with your metabolism and making you fatter and sicker by the minute. You may also be addicted to certain foods you probably didn't know were addictive. The way in which many food products are manufactured and marketed is compounding whatever personal issues you already have with food. Therefore I am going to make strong suggestions about what food you should *not* be eating if you want to achieve a healthy body composition and good overall health. But in the end it's up to you to decide what you choose to put in your mouth.

Eat to live. Don't live to eat.
Benjamin Franklin

Avoid Engineered Food

What passes for "food" these days? The truth is that food is being manufactured for profit, not for health. This goes beyond simply adding preservatives to ensure a long shelf life. Food companies are engineering food addiction by adding tasty chemicals such as MSG, unhealthy fats, and excessive amounts of salt, sugar, and artificial sweeteners.[15] Processed foods contain chemical substances that have been proven to create "addiction" in the consumer by stimulating the release of the same chemicals in your brain that certain types of drugs and alcohol do! Sugar has been likened to cocaine! The more a consumer is addicted to a certain food item, the more the manufacturer profits. Food manufacturers use the same business model that the tobacco companies used when they knowingly increased nicotine in their cigarettes to addict their customers and keep them coming back for more.

You could be eating to your heart's content. You could eat 10,000 calories a day and if you're not getting the specific nutrients your body needs in a way it can digest and assimilate, then you're starving on a nutritional basis, and as long as you're starving on a nutritional

basis, your body's going to stay hungry to get those
specific nutrients.

Weight-loss expert and author
Jon Gabriel, from *Food Matters*

High Calories, Low Nutrients

Most manufactured or highly processed foods have high calories and low nutritional value, which results in ongoing hunger, weight issues, and poor health. This relatively recent development poses an enormous threat to our population's overall well-being and quality of life. Weight gain, foggy thinking, headaches, and a lack of will to take self-responsibility are some of the milder symptoms of eating food with little or no nutritional value. Over the long term, eating highly processed foods on a regular basis can result in obesity, diabetes, heart disease, hormonal imbalance, and cancer. Diet foods, meal replacements, snack foods, breads, cereals, microwave meals, fast foods, and sodas (just to name a few) lack micronutrients, fiber, and phytochemicals—all of which are necessary if you want to maintain good overall health, high energy levels, and a stable, healthy weight.

Persuasive Marketing

Food manufacturers also use manipulating marketing strategies and tactics to lure us into buying unhealthy food products. I know firsthand the process that occurs when developing marketing campaigns for food products, in particular television commercials that manipulate people's psychology and areas of personal weakness. I once worked for a large soda company, and I'll also let you know that many of us did not consume the products we were advertising, because we knew what was inside them and that consuming them would *not* boost our self-esteem and confidence. We all know that advertising works. At one time or another, all of us have been enticed into buying a product because of a particularly provocative or appealing ad campaign. We are led to believe that certain "food" products, such as diet colas, will improve our health, appearance, sex appeal, or lifestyle, which will ultimately boost our confidence, desirability, and popularity. Ironically, the more we buy into the false claims, the more obese, sick, and depressed we get as a nation!

> *The marketing essentially lies to you, because it presents you with this image of a can of soda, and it doesn't tell you what's in the can. If you drink it, it's going to bring you these benefits by association—you're going to be cool, you're going to be sexy, you're going to be happy, you're going to be surrounded by friends, wearing skimpy bikinis or whatever their message happens to be . . . This is a lie. The truth is, if you drink that soda, you're going to lose bone mineral density because of the phosphoric acid it contains. If it's a diet soda, you may suffer neurological problems due to the chemical sweeteners, and if it's not a diet soda, it's probably made with high-fructose corn syrup, and that's going to promote type 2 diabetes and obesity.*
>
> Health journalist and author Mike Adams, from *Food Matters*

Skewed Studies

To make things much worse, food manufacturers have the power and financial backing to skew clinical studies in their favor. Consumers of processed foods are deceived and manipulated into buying unhealthy products, because they generally have little or no knowledge of the detrimental effects of all the additives listed on the product. Food companies conduct their own tests on the additives they want to use, and their advertising claims are often not verifiable.

Yet another physician who has seen these ill-health effects in his patients is Dr. Joseph Mercola, author and osteopathic physician:

> *Unfortunately, when a food additive like aspartame or any artificial sweetener is manufactured, the process of getting approval is really that the manufacturer, the company that's making it, is the one that funds the studies, and those are the studies that are submitted to the regulatory agency to provide approval. So it's not this independent third-party, objective evaluation that's being done.*[16]

Though I am personally outraged, mortified, and saddened by the information I am sharing with you, I also hope it's making you more aware of what's happening with our food. While we still need to recognize our responsibility and choice to change our health by making different choices, I also think it's of value for you to know what forces are out there working against your efforts. I encourage you to share this information with as many of your friends and family members as possible, in the hope we can collectively push back against these food manufacturers and withdraw our monetary support of their big business. By mass producing these so-called food products, designed to get us addicted so that we buy and consume more, they poison us and our children, and they make us fat and sick.

Bad Foods Zap Our Life Force

Just think back to when you last ate something natural and clean, like an organic apple picked directly from the tree. Remember how good it made you feel physically, mentally, spiritually, and emotionally? When a food is in its fully natural form, it is rich in nutrients and a natural energy source that our bodies are *meant* to consume. Now recall the last time you inhaled a processed pizza, a big family-size bag of potato chips, a large serving of fries, or a packet of candy at the cinema. How did you feel after eating those foods? Lousy—am I right? Or perhaps you can no longer tell the difference because it's been so long that you've consumed anything that's sugar free, organic, and nutrient dense. That's because these phony "foods" actually rob us of our energy. These foods are not really foods at all; they are simply sugary food "products," with little to no nutritional value, dressed up in disguise.

Every single human being on this planet deserves to be nourished and energized by natural foods produced by an earth that belongs to the whole of humanity, not just a few companies. Fortunately, we still have a plentiful supply of the natural foods that can provide us all the nutritional value we need for an energetic, abundant life. We need a better understanding of how our food is produced, so we can choose the best food for our health and our bodies. We may have to fight for it, but the choices we make when we are shopping for our family's food can send a powerful message to food manufacturing companies:

we know what is good for us because we are listening to our bodies, not their advertising!

Eat the *Right* Fat to Lose Weight and Maintain Health

Dietary fat is a somewhat controversial subject these days. There are different types of fat, and it is generally acknowledged by everyone that trans fats (also known as hydrogenated fats) are unhealthy, while unsaturated fats (monounsaturated and polyunsaturated) have huge health benefits. In fact, polyunsaturated fats found in foods like salmon, almond butter, hemp, and flaxseed are necessary for the healthy functioning of the entire body. So, yes, there is such a thing as a "healthy fat."

You may be surprised to learn that "fat free" can actually be more "fattening" than healthy fat itself. How? Foods that claim to be "fat free" replace dietary fat with excessive amounts of sugar to boost flavor. When the body takes in more sugar than it can use, the sugar gets metabolized by the body and stored as fat on the body! So while fat is not technically contained within the product, it still makes your body produce fat. Some examples of unhealthy, "fat-free" foods that are really loaded with sugar include milk, yogurts, and cereals.

It's vitally important for you to eat healthy dietary fats to support your body's proper functioning and overall health. Healthy dietary fats, along with protein, help you feel satiated, which naturally prevents you from craving more food and thus lose weight or maintain a healthy weight.

Both monounsaturated and polyunsaturated fats are also thought to have beneficial effects on cholesterol levels. Polyunsaturated fats are a good source of omega-3 fatty acids, which have been shown to support brain function, reduce inflammation, and possibly lower the risk of diseases such as cancer, heart disease, bipolar disorder, and arthritis.

A deficiency of omega-3 fatty acids can lead to poor circulation, heart problems, joint pain, dry skin, brittle hair, fatigue, impaired memory, and depression. Some good food sources of omega-3 fatty acids include salmon, shrimp, walnuts, flaxseeds, cabbage, tuna, mackerel, oregano, anchovies, scallops, cauliflower, kale, brussels sprouts, halibut, cod, soybeans, tofu, and collard greens. Good, healthy sources of monounsaturated fats are found in peanuts, cashews, extra virgin olive oil, almonds, pecans, pistachios, canola oil, avocados, and sesame oil.

As a result of food label laws, "trans fats" are listed on all packaged foods, although the FDA allows manufacturers to put "0 trans fats" labels on anything with 0. 5 grams or fewer of trans fat per serving. Small amounts of trans fats occur naturally in lamb, beef, and full-fat dairy products, but most trans fats are artificially created fats made during a hydrogenation process in which liquid vegetable oil is converted into solid fat.

Trans fats have been used in processed foods to prolong a product's shelf life and can still be found (often listed as partially hydrogenated vegetable oil) in packaged cookies, crackers, cakes, muffins, hamburger buns, margarine, vegetable shortening, cake mixes, pancake mixes, fried foods, donuts, French fries, chicken nuggets, hard taco shells, chips, candy, microwave popcorn, and frozen dinners. Trans fats are considered to be unhealthy because they: 1) raise bad cholesterol, and 2) lower good cholesterol. Studies have found that they increase our risk of heart disease, obesity, and obesity-related diseases such as diabetes.

Non-organic sources of fat of all types are also often damaging. Research has shown that fats that have been altered by oxygen, heat, and industrial farming practices can cause a build-up of plaque on the walls of the blood vessels, which can then contribute to heart disease and other serious illnesses. Damaged or rancid fats can be found in pasteurized dairy products, meats that have been deep fried, most vegetable oils, and all hydrogenated oils.

As far as we know, saturated fats can be good to a point, but should be eaten in moderation.[17] Saturated fats are found in meat, eggs, cheese, butter, cream, and palm and coconut oils and are an important source of vitamins and minerals. Many scientists and health-care professionals believe too much saturated fat is dangerous and can cause heart disease and diabetes, but there are dissenting voices that claim just the opposite. Some studies have shown that a diet high in saturated fat can benefit people with type 2 diabetes and can actually protect against cardiovascular disease. It has also been said by some that a diet high in saturated fat is good for bone strength, can boost the immune system, can fight and prevent cancer, and can improve liver, lung, brain, and nerve function. The scientists and researchers who advocate diets high in saturated fat are adamant that all sources of saturated fat be organic.

Avoid Harmful Additives

Monosodium glutamate (MSG) is probably the most well-known food additive. Glutamate is a naturally occurring, non-essential (meaning the body can produce it on its own) amino acid that influences your ability to detect and taste savory flavors. It also has an impact on the central nervous system. We generally consume a moderate (safe) amount of naturally occurring glutamate when we eat certain vegetable and animal proteins. MSG is glutamate combined with sodium. It's added to food to enhance the savory flavor of processed items such as gravy, stuffing, sauce, crackers, and luncheon meat. MSG is considered a flavor enhancer, not a food additive, and so is not regulated as an additive.

For some people, eating food with added MSG can temporarily cause headaches, nausea, a burning sensation, and chest pains. In highly sensitive people, high doses of MSG may, over time, cause neurological problems, as high doses of glutamate can act as a neurotoxin. If these possible side effects don't put you off MSG, consider the fact that it causes obesity in lab rats and is routinely used for that purpose. According to experts, MSG is apparently in 80 percent of all flavored foods, and it activates chemicals in the brain that *increase* fat gain and obesity.

Another FDA-approved additive is *propylene glycol C3H8O2.* Propylene glycol is made from petroleum and is an odorless, clear liquid deemed by the FDA to be safe that is used to keep foods moist and stabilized. It is also injected into live cattle to prevent them from losing fat. Some of the processed foods that contain propylene glycol are fast-food burgers, salad dressing, chips, ice cream, soy sauce, soda, yogurt, juice, and blueberry muffins. According to the documentary *Food Matters,* the "blueberries" you find in your commercially made muffins are made from propylene glycol, partially hydrogenated oils, liquid sugar, and artificial color. They are not even real blueberries! In addition to being used as an additive/preservative in the foods we eat, propylene glycol is also commonly used as antifreeze. Now, isn't that a pleasant thought?

Avoid Sugar: Excess Refined Sugar Produces Fat Cells

One of the primary reasons most overweight people are overweight is because they eat too much refined sugar. This may seem obvious, but the amount of refined sugar you can consume in a day, even if you are not eating candy, cookies, or cake, is astounding if you are not paying attention. Some form of refined sugar is added to almost all packaged, processed, or pre-prepared foods, as well as canned and bottled beverages. I use the term "refined sugar" to distinguish the sugar added to packaged and processed foods and beverages from the naturally occurring, healthy sugars in fruits, dairy, vegetables, and some grains. So how much sugar should we be eating?

Naturally occurring sugars are good for us and an essential part of a healthy diet. Refined sugar, on the other hand, has been linked to a variety of diseases, such as obesity, diabetes, tooth decay, cancer, and heart disease. The American Heart Association's guidelines for refined sugar intake are no more than 100 calories (about 6 teaspoons) a day for most women and no more than 150 calories (about 9 teaspoons) a day for most men.[18] The majority of Americans consume more than 355 calories (22 teaspoons) of refined sugar a day. And what does the body do with that excess sugar?

> Once the [excess] sugar is ingested, it will turn into fat in the body. Why? Because it sends the sugar levels sky high. And what does the pancreas do? It has to secrete insulin in order to bring that down so you don't die. Insulin is the fat-producing hormone. So all this excess energy comes along [in the form of sugar] and [the body] says, where can we store it? Short-term places, liver . . . but what do we do with the excess? I know what we'll do. We'll produce some fat cells . . .

Author and addiction specialist Jason Vale, from *Food Matters*

There are many different names for sugar (over one hundred, in fact), and some of them are intended to dupe us into buying them because they "sound" so harmless. But remember, armed with knowledge, we can choose to avoid all forms of refined sugar, or consume it in moderation, knowing exactly what sugar does to our bodies. Avoiding processed and packaged foods is the way to go.

Listed in alphabetical order are just some of the names for sugar you might find in the ingredients list on packaged and processed foods and beverages: barley malt, beet sugar, brown sugar, cane-juice crystals, cane sugar, caramel, carob syrup, confectioner's sugar, corn sweetener, corn syrup, corn syrup solids, date sugar, dextran, dextrose, diatase, diastatic malt, ethyl maltol, fructose, fruit juice, fruit juice concentrate, galactose, glucose, glucose solids, golden sugar, grape sugar, granulated sugar, high-fructose corn syrup (or HFCS), honey, invert sugar, juice, lactose, malt syrup, maltodextrin, maltose, mannitol, maple sugar, maple syrup, molasses, raw sugar, refiner's syrup, sorbitol, sorghum syrup, sucrose, syrup, and turbinado sugar. (To get more names for sugar, visit my blog at www. MichelleArmstrong.com.)

Artificial Sweeteners Can Be Deadly

High-fructose corn syrup is basically a very cheaply manufactured, highly refined sugar syrup extracted from corn (corn growers in the United States get enormous subsidies from the government), very similar to white cane or beet sugar. It can be found anywhere you might find sugar and is often added along with sugar to jam, juice, cookies, cake, candy, bread, frosting, ice cream, ketchup, tomato sauce, and luncheon meat. Not only does it make everything sweeter, but it also acts as a preservative and can extend the shelf life of a product by years!

High-fructose corn syrup causes all of the same health problems that sugar does, including increased risk of heart disease, obesity, poor immunity, diabetes, anemia, elevated LDL (bad) cholesterol, and tooth decay.

If you are wondering whether any artificial sweeteners are safe, the answer is not a simple one. There is a tremendous amount of inconclusive and conflicting information on artificial sweeteners, due to the fact that the companies producing the sweeteners are often the ones who conduct the research and set up the studies to determine whether or not they are safe. There are, however, independent studies that show evidence of cancer in lab animals who have consumed large quantities of artificial sweeteners, and a wide variety of reports from consumers claiming to have experienced medical conditions ranging from headaches and nausea, to multiple sclerosis, fibromyalgia, and seizures as a result of ingesting artificial sweeteners. There is also scientific evidence that some artificial sweeteners actually *cause* weight gain.

Low- or no-calorie artificial sweeteners, such as aspartame, saccharine, sucralose, neotame, and acesulfame K (also known as acesulfame potassium, Ace-K, or Sunett) are routinely used as alternatives to sugar. These sweeteners can be found in a huge variety of products, such as nutritional bars, flavored waters, fruit spreads, cereals, breath mints, juice blends, meal replacements, iced tea, chewing gum, and soft drinks, just to name a few. And, depending on what they are combined with, artificial sweeteners can prove deadly. Here's what Christiane Northrup, MD, has to say about the "deadly" combination of caffeine and aspartame in diet colas: "Nothing else does it in your brain quite like a diet cola. And that's because there's a deadly combination there of aspartame and caffeine, and those two together create a very unique blend of excitotoxins that kill off brain cells. But before they die, they have this excitement that's like a buzz."[19]

Food for thought: Did you know that airline pilots don't drink diet sodas, because it's well recognized within the Pilots Association that drinking diet soda can cause a severe vision aberration that can potentially lead to problems with their flying?

Consuming "Empty" Calories Creates a High-Calorie Diet

Empty-calorie foods are high-calorie, processed food-like substances that contain unhealthy fats, sugars, artificial sweeteners, salt, and other additives and preservatives. These foods are not empty of calories—they are empty of nutritional value. They do not contain the macro- and micronutrients needed by the body to maintain optimal health and well-being (see Appendix B, Nutrition Basics, for more about the macro- and micronutrients our bodies need). The extra calories consumed in empty-calorie foods are stored in the body as fat, will most likely result in weight gain, and may ultimately result in obesity and debilitating and/or life-threatening disease.

Nutrient-Dense Foods Decrease Hunger and Food Cravings

Nutrient-dense foods provide more nutrients than calories, while empty-calorie foods contain more calories than nutrients. Nutrient-dense foods include unprocessed organic fruits and vegetables, nuts, whole grains, raw dairy products, seeds, beans, fish, and organic meats. These foods provide macronutrients and micronutrients, such as vitamins, minerals, amino acids, healthy dietary fats, essential fatty acids, and healthy carbohydrates, and may help reduce the incidence of heart disease, diabetes, and cancer. The high-fiber content and healthy fats in nutrient-dense foods also makes you feel satiated, which means you will be less inclined to overeat. "In my experience treating thousands of patients and guiding them through transitioning to a high-nutrient-density diet," says Joel Fuhrman, MD, "I have observed that my patients' perceptions of hunger change. As their diet improves, feelings of hunger become less frequent, less uncomfortable . . . ."[20]

Eating Organic Foods Satiates the Body's Cravings

Simply put, "organic" foods are foods made naturally by Mother Earth and not in a lab room. The body was designed to consume natural foods, perfectly created by the beauty of life, not by a scientist in a petri dish!

I know the term "organic" is becoming a buzzword these days, and its definition is quietly being eroded by food manufacturers for their own personal gain. Let's clarify the meaning of the term by using the US Department of Agriculture's (USDA's) definition of what constitutes organic food:

Organic food is produced by farmers who emphasize the use of renewable resources and the conservation of soil and water to enhance environmental quality for future generations. Organic meat, poultry, eggs, and dairy products come from animals that are given no antibiotics or growth hormones. Organic food is produced without using most conventional pesticides; fertilizers made with synthetic ingredients or sewage sludge; bioengineering; or ionizing radiation. Before a product can be labeled "organic," a government-approved certifier inspects the farm where the food is grown to make sure the farmer is following all the rules necessary to meet USDA organic standards. Companies that handle or process organic food before it gets to your local supermarket or restaurant must be certified too.[21]

Organic foods—fruits and vegetables, meat and dairy—not only taste a thousand times better than non-organic foods, but they have higher nutritional value. The nutrients severely lacking in many people's diets are precisely the vitamins and minerals that organic food offers us. When we eat lots of packaged and processed food and still crave more, we are not craving the refined sugars, damaged fats, additives, and chemicals that are often made to look and taste like natural food. The body is actually crying out for the real nutrients it needs to thrive. When we deprive our body of these essentials, we are starving ourselves, even as we get fatter!

Food for Thought

Most experts agree with the general verdicts covered above: avoid processed foods, and eat food as close to its natural state as possible for maximum health. However, as you well know, there are many more controversial topics regarding food where established experts—scientists, medical doctors, nutritionists, and wellness practitioners—offer directly opposing advice! So even though I may have strong opinions about some of the topics below, they are my own, based on my own research, knowledge, experience, and best judgment. I'd encourage you to do what I did: keep researching, keep checking in with your own body, and make the decision that's right for you.

Genetically Modified Foods

Genetically modified (GM) foods have been subjected to genetic engineering, whereby certain genes are inserted into a plant or animal to achieve a specific result. These are scientists playing God, in my opinion, with little regard for the impact they're making on human lives. This is different from the older, slower method of genetic modification through selective breeding, in which a plant or animal that exhibits a desirable trait is favored in the planting or breeding process until the desired trait shows up more consistently. This process has been employed for centuries and has never been considered unsafe.

Typically, GM grains are genetically modified to increase resistance to herbicides and pesticides, so that when these toxins are sprayed to eliminate weeds and bugs, the crops are not harmed. GM food producers claim that GM foods produce higher crop yields and have the potential to eliminate hunger worldwide. There is still no evidence of this, I might add. According to the World Food Programme, 870 million people in the world do not have enough to eat. Up to 70 percent of processed/packaged foods in the US contain genetically modified ingredients, which, as of this writing, are not required to be disclosed in package labeling. The most common foods to be genetically modified are corn, soybeans, and grapeseed oil. GM grains are also routinely used in animal feed.

Some claim GM foods are safe for human consumption. I wholeheartedly disagree with this claim, because there is too much evidence that people are experiencing negative side effects, such as liver and kidney damage and lowered immune responses, from eating GM foods. In the US, these foods are not required by the government to be assessed for safety. Some countries around the world have banned GM foods, but plenty of other countries have embraced the GM trend and no countries conduct adequate long-term safety tests. Many "safety" tests are conducted by the companies that produce these foods, so the test results cannot be trusted, in my opinion. I invite you to continue to research GM foods and make your own decisions about whether or not you feel comfortable eating them.

Meat

When it comes to consuming meat, the choice is fully up to you, since there are so many opposing arguments on the subject. Meat is an excellent source of protein for the body, but it's not the only protein source. If you do eat meat, I would ask you to consider if the meat you're consuming is good for you and if the animals you're consuming are receiving the level of humane treatment that all of God's creatures deserve. Personally, I only eat organic chicken and fish, since I believe we become what we eat, and because I am mortified and deeply saddened by the treatment of many animals at large meat manufacturing plants and farms. But I am also strongly considering becoming a vegan or vegetarian, and I continue to research and pray about this lifestyle change. I recommend that if you eat meat, you only eat organic meats. But you need to decide what feels right for you.

In my research on meat production for this book, I learned sadly that many of today's factory farm animals are being treated inhumanely, to say the very least. They are often crammed into tiny spaces and cages by the thousands and forced to live in filthy, windowless conditions. They don't get to experience the grass beneath their feet, sunlight on their skins, or breathe fresh air until they are loaded onto the trucks that transport them to their slaughter. Before they are slaughtered, they are fed drugs to fatten them up faster and keep them alive in conditions that would otherwise kill them. Just imagine walking a mile in their animal's shoes – my heart feels as though it's breaking in two when I do.

Can you fathom that in some countries, dolphin meat is on the menu? Dolphins are kind, gentle, sentient beings with a greater level of intelligence, emotional sensitivity, and awareness than humans. At a place called The Cove in Taiji, Japan, thousands of dolphins every year are brutally, barbarically, and inhumanely tortured and slaughtered for their meat—which is not even healthy for human consumption due to its high mercury content. The reason for the slaughter and production of unhealthy meat? Greed. I don't know about you, but I certainly do not want to be partaking in the consumption of animals that are treated with such cruelty and disrespect. As I mentioned earlier, I'm not sure I want to continue the consumption of animals at all. But this is personal consideration and we are each entitled to our choices. These creatures nourish and fuel *our* bodies, and this is the treatment and thanks we give them? Unacceptable, in my opinion. The stress these animals undergo is not only unthinkable and inhumane, but the stress, suffering, and pain they carry in their bodies, you then eat and put in yours.

Dairy

It may seem counterintuitive, but according to some food experts, pasteurized dairy products are bad for you. They draw our attention instead to the many health benefits that can result from consuming unpasteurized, unhomogenized, raw dairy products from grass-fed cows. Raw milk, straight from the cow, is a living, complete food—it contains every essential amino acid, healthy carbohydrates, healthy amounts of necessary saturated fat, healthy amounts of necessary cholesterol, and a complete array of bio-available vitamins, minerals, enzymes, and beneficial bacteria. Before pasteurization was a common practice, raw milk was often used medicinally because of all the beneficial nutrients it contains. It has been said to boost the immune system, aid in digestion, provide resistance from many bacteria and viruses, reduce the incidence of certain cancers, improve bone density, regulate hormones, and reduce the risk of heart disease.

On the other hand, according to the United States' FDA website, "Raw milk can harbor dangerous microorganisms that can pose a serious health risk to you and your family." The pasteurization process heats milk to a specific temperature in order to kill the germs that cause salmonella and E. coli. But when you look at the big picture, pasteurization is not a purely beneficial process. Pasteurization also kills or destroys most of the beneficial nutrients in raw milk, and it makes it undrinkable for those with lactose intolerance, as the enzymes in raw milk allow even those with lactose intolerance to digest it. Pasteurizing raw milk also makes it dangerous to consume. The heat damages the fat in the milk, making it more likely to cause a build-up of plaque on the walls of the blood vessels, which can then contribute to heart disease and other serious illnesses. Finally, pasteurization renders most of the natural, bio-available calcium in raw milk insoluble, so it is no longer available to the body and does not contribute to bone health, despite the continued claims by the mainstream milk industry. For more information on milk, see Appendix B.

Wheat

Before I developed a greater awareness of my body, I used to eat a lot of wheat— breads and pastas in particular. But when I began listening to my body, I realized it was sending signs that it was rejecting wheat. I observed an increase in feelings of fatigue, brain-fog, forgetfulness, weight gain, and feelings of depression that occurred only when I ate wheat; I knew intuitively it wasn't right for my body. While I haven't omitted wheat completely from my diet, I now eat very little. I have included whole-wheat products on my suggested food list at the end of this chapter, as have I meat, since it's a personal preference and not my place to mandate but rather to expand awareness, but I encourage you to follow your intuition, do some more research, pay more intimate attention to your body, pray, and/or meditate about it, and then arrive at your own conclusion about whether to include wheat in your diet. My recommendation is to ditch wheat where possible and get your complex carbohydrates in the form of vegetables and alternate grains such as quinoa, amaranth, buckwheat, raw organic oats, and sweet potato.

According to William Davis, MD, author of *Wheat Belly*, many of the wheat-based products we consume, such as whole-wheat bread, muffins, and bagels, are having a detrimental effect on our bodies and could be the cause of health problems such as fatigue, gastrointestinal distress, obesity, diabetes, inflammation, and unwanted belly fat. According to Dr. Davis, certain wheat products can increase blood sugar levels to those *higher* than sugar.

In an interview with Dr. Davis on the website Macleans.ca, he asserts that most wheat is genetically modified and that its "safety for human consumption has never been tested or questioned." He goes on to say that organic whole wheat is really not significantly better for you and that eliminating wheat altogether is really the only route to better health and a healthy weight. Wheat contains a carbohydrate (amylopectin A) "which is more efficiently converted to blood sugar than just about any other carbohydrate, including table sugar." In other words, you will experience the same high you get from eating a candy bar and the same crash, which will then prompt you to eat more in order to get your energy back—it's a vicious cycle. Eating wheat products throughout the day will leave you, as Dr. Davis says, "constantly feeling hungry and constantly eating." He points out that if you eliminate wheat from your diet, you won't feel hungry between meals and will find that you lose weight much more easily and quickly than you would if you were to continue eating wheat.

If I haven't convinced you to reduce or give up bread and pasta yet, I encourage you to ponder the following quote from the interview with Dr. Davis:

> Small low-density lipoprotein (LDL) particles form when you're eating lots of carbohydrates, and they are responsible for atherosclerotic plaque, which in turn triggers heart disease and stroke. So even if you're a slender, vigorous, healthy person, you're still triggering the formation of small

LDL particles. And second, carbohydrates increase your blood sugars, which cause this process of glycation, that is, the glucose modification of proteins. If I glycate the proteins in my eyes, I get cataracts. If I glycate the cartilage of my knees and hips, I get arthritis. If I glycate small LDL, I'm more prone to atherosclerosis. So it's a twofold effect. And if you don't start out slender and keep eating that fair trade, organically grown whole wheat bread that sounds so healthy, you're repeatedly triggering high blood sugars and are going to wind up with more visceral fat. This isn't just what I call the wheat belly that you can see, flopping over your belt, but the fat around your internal organs. And as visceral fat accumulates, you risk responses like diabetes and heart disease.

I encourage you to visit Dr. Davis' blog for more information at www.wheatbellyblog.com.

Juice

While there are some small benefits to juice cleanses, the general consensus is that long-term juicing isn't good for your health and is not the best pathway to losing weight. I have witnessed this in my studio—juicing results in short-term weight loss that doesn't last long-term. The key is always a little of everything in moderation.

On the other hand, replacing one meal a day with a fruit or vegetable blend—where you process the whole fruit or vegetable in your blender to retain the fiber—is deemed acceptable as long it is supported with a complete and balanced diet. That means enough portions of fresh fruit and vegetables in unblended form, natural whole grains, and lean organic sources of protein. I also prefer vegetables blends as opposed to fruit blends, since fruits contain natural sugars, and too much sugar, whether natural or not, can be detrimental to weight loss and a healthy body composition. But since fruits are so rich in antioxidants, consuming one fruit a day in blended form can be enormously beneficial to your health. So again, I invite you to be the judge by observing how your own body responds and to pray and meditate on it.

I also suggest that if you're going to juice, juice green vegetables and not loads of fruits to avoid consuming too much sugar. Juicing your veggies once a day can also be beneficial if you find you are not great at consuming an adequate amount of vegetables per day for healthy living, or if you have a very busy schedule and time is of the essence.

Juicing can provide a wonderful way to detox and cleanse every now and again. I like to detox and cleanse my body two to three times a year. But I don't juice straight all day long and *never* for longer than two to three days. Instead I focus on eliminating all foods high in toxins and increase my water, vegetable, and fruit consumption. I also never include more than one piece of fruit in my juices. If you're going to juice for the purpose of detoxing and cleansing, I suggest making it short and *not* sweet. It's simply not healthy to restrict the other nutrients your body needs from other foods. Juicing might be faster and easier than making a meal, but if your lifestyle requires you to juice your foods for the sake of time, I suggest looking at and making some changes to your lifestyle. If you don't have time to make a healthy meal, then your life is far too busy. Instead of juicing to improve your health, I suggest slowing your life down to make time for your health and healthier meals.

Surprisingly, juicing can actually be dangerous for some of us. One *Huffington Post* article indicates that an ongoing diet of juicing can leave your body without necessary macronutrients, such as fats, which can contribute to the malabsorption of fat-soluble vitamins and proteins, which are responsible for the building of new tissue.[22] Because of the high sugar content of many juices, juicing can also be dangerous for diabetics and people with kidney disease or undergoing chemotherapy. The article states: "Because juice doesn't offer the fiber contained in fruits and veggies, the body absorbs fructose sugar more easily, which can affect blood sugar levels, according to Food Republic. If you do decide to try a juice cleanse, drink more veggie juices and limit fruit juice to one glass a day in order to avoid this potential side effect."[23] Juicing also produces the side effect of loose bowels and/or diarrhea, and can create cravings due to the low caloric value and low fat content—which may result in short-term weight loss, but will ultimately result in putting the weight straight back on almost immediately.

Let me put it this way—because of the high sugar content, juice drinks and juice boxes have been banned from many schools, just as soda has been. Juice is not allowed at the school my son attends. I am thrilled!

Listen to Your Body

The simplest and best way to eat is as follows: Eat in moderation. Eat smaller, regular meals throughout the day. Eat clean, organic, and fresh. And when the experts disagree and you aren't sure whether a particular food is good for you or not, you have a wonderful opportunity to learn the most important lesson of all: listen to your own body. The best way I know how to do that is to mediate and pray, and *eat mindfully.*

What do I mean by mindfully? Whenever you eat, you can eat mindfully simply by choosing to fully experience what you're eating and not rush the nourishing process. Eat each piece of food slowly and with abundant gratitude. Observe when you have reached a comfortable level of satiety and don't feel the need to continue eating. Are you *aware* of what it actually feels like to be comfortably full from eating? Can you tell the difference between true hunger and toxic or emotional hunger? Become aware of the colour of your food. Notice its texture, smell, taste, and viscosity in your mouth. You may not be eating mindfully, and so this particular practice will be of great value to you.

While some studies suggest some people are physically unable to determine when they are full due to chemical processes within the brain, I believe even this situation is rectifiable through mindfulness and awareness. We can develop the ability to be mindfully aware and deeply connected to our body *if* we give it our attention and presence. Again, meditation and prayer can help with this. After all, listening to our body is completely natural. We know how to listen and respond to it when it informs us that we need to sleep, go to the bathroom, or put on a sweater when it's cold. There is no reason why we can't tune into the body for information about when to stop eating and what to eat. We probably lost some of that intrinsic skill when processed foods with addictive additives were introduced into our diets. But we also lost it when we stopped paying attention to our mental, emotional, spiritual, and physical bodies – when we stopped being present, quiet and still.

If you find that you are indeed hungry, ask your awareness what food your body needs right now. Is it an apple (a complex carbohydrate), a piece of turkey (protein), or some avocado or nut butter (a healthy fat)? Is it water? Are you dehydrated? When you can become intimately aware of and connected to your body, you will easily be able to discern between true physical hunger and emotional need. Cultivate your body awareness along with your food knowledge. These are significant steps towards overcoming food addiction. It will take time and practice, but you can eventually achieve this mind-body mastery.

If you pay attention to when you are hungry, what your body wants, what you are eating, when you've had enough, you end the obsession, because obsession and awareness cannot coexist.

Geneen Roth

I don't follow the philosophy of strict calorie counting as I don't believe it's necessary nor natural, and I don't believe there is one perfect diet for everybody. Instead of adhering to a specific type of diet, I encourage you to eat mindfully, and to create your own unique diet based on how your body, mood, and energy levels respond to what *you* eat and when you eat it. Mindful eating is not a diet strategy—it is a way to bring awareness to every aspect of eating. By slowing down enough to observe the color, texture, aroma, and flavor of your food, you are able to observe yourself, your emotions, your sensations, and your reactions as you eat. Eating mindfully eliminates the inclination to overeat, improves digestion, enhances your enjoyment of food, and produces feelings of genuine satisfaction.

When you eat, begin to notice if there are any changes that occur in your physical body. Do you experience any stiffness, tingling, bloating, cramping, nausea, or diarrhea? Notice what happens to you emotionally. Do you find that suddenly you feel depressed, giddy, stressed, anxious, forgetful, agitated, or impatient? Does your perception or focus change at all as a result of what you eat? If you eat something and feel very pleasantly satiated and don't have any negative physical or emotional responses—if anything, you feel more energized, more aware, more present—then that food is probably good for you.

Sometimes you will find that you can eat certain foods, like oatmeal and blueberries, in the morning without a problem, but if you eat that same meal in the afternoon, you get a completely different psychological and physical response. When you're premenstrual or when you're going through different hormonal phases in life, what you can eat and enjoy will change. What you can eat in your twenties might be different from what you can eat in your forties. So you see that this process of determining what foods are best for you is ongoing. You will become more and more sensitive to what feels right for your body, and you will start to automatically change your food choices as a result. In my personal experience I can pick up a food and just by holding it close, can tune into its energy and know intuitively whether or not that food is right for my body and at that moment.

If you are not used to cooking for yourself, I encourage you to learn to shop, prepare, and cook your own food. You don't have to become a master chef; (I certainly am not) I just want you to develop a healthy, respectful, and loving relationship with your food, even if it's as simple as planning and preparing a garden salad. I am personally not very creative in the kitchen at all. But by becoming more involved with my food, I am learning to love being in the kitchen, and I enjoy finding new and exciting (albeit easy) recipes. By being fully responsible and fully involved in your own transformation, you create a greater opportunity for lasting success.

Awareness Transforms Addiction

In his book *Overcoming Addiction*, Deepak Chopra says, "Awareness, intention, mindfulness, and learning to focus on the inner intelligence of your body as well as the supreme wisdom of the universe, which expresses itself in you, are the guiding principles of healthy eating."[24] No one can tell you how much you should weigh or how much you should eat. You really know these things intuitively yourself. You just need to become aware of your body's inner wisdom.

To awaken this awareness and mindfulness, Chopra suggests that before you begin to eat, you place your hand on your belly to assess your hunger level and tune into what your stomach is really telling you. Is your belly really hungry? Or is the desire for food coming from another need? Is it truly ice cream or a bowl of creamy pasta? Or do you actually need to feel safe, calm, and loved? Literally ask your body, then answer yourself.

In his article "Redefining Hunger Can Kick Start Weight Loss," Joel Fuhrman, MD, explains the difference between the healthy hunger that comes from your body communicating its needs, and the toxic hunger you experience when your stomach growls and you feel irritable, tired, and spaced out. When you feel "toxic hunger," you are not experiencing "true" hunger, but rather withdrawal from the toxic high-calorie, non-nutritive, pre-prepared, packaged, processed junk foods you are used to eating. Eating more unhealthy food to eliminate these uncomfortable feelings of "hunger" just perpetuates the cycle of overeating, which "has led to an epidemic of obesity, and a continual rise in preventable chronic diseases."[25]

Dr. Fuhrman goes on to propose that eating a healthy, nutrient-rich diet will eliminate the uncomfortable withdrawal symptoms you now associate with hunger pains. Instead of the daily experience of being unfocused, grouchy, and tired, you will feel "true hunger" when you are naturally ready to eat again. He characterizes true hunger as feelings "mainly felt in the mouth and throat." He explains that you will feel hungry less frequently, and those feelings will be less uncomfortable than the "toxic hunger" you feel when you are eating junk food.[26]

Recently a client shared with me how great she felt as a result of removing wheat, dairy, and sugar from her diet. Before removing those foods from her diet, she described herself as feeling: "ugh, heavy, bloated, lethargic, unable to think clearly, depressed, sad, irritable, anxious, and generally unwell." Now she feels like a brand-new woman who has clarity of thought and feels relaxed, calm, and "lighter" in her body. She no longer feels hungry all the time, she has heaps more energy, and depression and anxiety are things of the past.

What we eat affects us physically, emotionally, mentally, and spiritually. As we transition into my specific food guidelines, I invite you to write down how you feel *before* you start following my guidelines, so you can look back in a few weeks and compare how you *feel* as a result of following the guidelines. I know when I cut out wheat, dairy, red meat, and sugar, I felt a thousand times better. I am a person who rarely takes any sort of medication, and I believe this has a great deal to do with the source of my nutrition—real food—which is the best medicine to improve health and wellness. When you've hit on the right balance for you, your body will let you know with its vibrancy and clarity.

Nutritional Guidelines

Now that you know more about what is happening to your food, you can make empowered and educated decisions and choices from this point on. To achieve a new level of wellness and a healthy body composition and maintain or achieve your ideal physique, all you need to do now is follow these simple guidelines and your goals will easily be made manifest. When it comes to nutrition, I like to keep things very simple, which is why I have created for you a set of guidelines as well as a list of what to eat and what not to eat for the purpose of achieving a healthy body composition. The guidelines provided are what I follow on a daily basis and what I encourage my clients to follow as well. These guidelines have, time and time again, transformed bodies and lives for the better. They are healthy and they work. However, I invite you to be responsible for your own health and body and encourage you to conduct your own research on what you choose to put in your mouth. I suggest you apply these 18 simple guidelines as soon as possible and monitor and track your results. Experience, not words or even research studies, will prove to you what's best for *your* unique and precious body long term. Remember to always consult your medical physician before embarking on new nutrition programs, including this one.

1. Eat smaller meals more often. Eat approximately every 3 hours, so that you eat 4—6 meals a day, depending on your lifestyle and activity. Listen to your body and monitor what it needs as you explore this new rhythm.

2. Manage your portions.

I am a better person when I have less on my plate.
Elizabeth Gilbert, *Eat, Pray, Love*

Most of us are eating far too much food at one sitting, while not eating often enough throughout the day. . People who come to my studio often tell me that they eat nothing during the day except perhaps a coffee or maybe a piece of fruit or a yogurt. They then have a giant meal at dinnertime, when they come home from work starving to death because they've deprived their bodies of nutrients all day.

For appropriate serving sizes of the macronutrients—fats, carbs, and proteins—for your unique body and goals, speak with a registered holistic nutritionist or dietician.

3. Create your meals from the "Eat These Foods" list and avoid all items on the "Avoid These Foods" list found at the end of this chapter.

4. Eat breakfast *every day* without fail and within 30 minutes of waking. Breakfast should be your *largest* meal of the day—approximately 25–35% of your overall daily caloric intakes—and should absolutely include all the necessary meal elements shown on the plate: proteins, complex carbs, and healthy fats. It is also advantageous to consume the majority of your daily carbohydrate allowance *prior* to exercise or major activity. If at night after work you tend to be sedentary, then it can be beneficial to omit certain carbohydrates like starchy carbohydrates altogether.

5. Stick to just 1–2 servings of fruit per day. Remember that fruit is sugar, and if you need to lose body fat, be conscious of your fruit (sugar) consumption. For those seeking to lose weight, I suggest just 1 piece of fruit per day, preferably in the mornings or after your workouts, until you've achieved your desired body composition.

6. Omit all dairy where possible. We've all heard that dairy is a good source of protein, calcium, vitamin D, and vitamin B12. However, according to some nutritional experts, most people are allergic to dairy, and you can easily get all the nutrients you need from a variety of clean and healthy foods. I invite you to pay attention and listen to what your body needs. Omitting dairy is not mandatory, but I do suggest taking it out of your diet for a few weeks to observe what happens in your body and to notice how you feel. Then if you want to reintroduce it, consider eating dairy only 2–3 times a week and adhere to a portion side of 1/2–1 cup. If you do omit dairy completely, I recommend consulting with a registered dietician to learn how to replace the nutrients dairy provides with non-dairy substitutes. Also be sure to avoid the known "calcium thieves," such as salt, alcohol, caffeine, and a sedentary lifestyle.

7. **One to two meals can be replaced with a protein smoothie, if desired.** If you live a busy lifestyle, a smoothie is a fast, efficient way to get in your daily nutrients. Avoid using more than one piece of fruit in your smoothies to avoid consuming too much sugar, and add vegetables to shakes for added nutritional value. Whey protein or plant protein is fine. I personally use a combination of both. You just need to ensure your protein source meets the recommended serving size. Ideally use your shake meals for after your strength training workouts (see chapter 11) to replenish, heal, and repair your muscles.

8. **Consume from the low to medium end of the Glycemic Index if fat loss is your goal.** However, after a good strength training workout, a healthy and natural high GI food in combination with your protein source can be beneficial to support the body's rapid absorption of the protein to your muscles. A protein shake after a workout is a great example.

9. **Limit sodium intake to approximate 1500 mg a day.** If that proves difficult, 2300 mg may be a more manageable goal, as recommended by the USDA Dietary Reference Intakes, and will still produce health benefits.

10. **Ensure adequate consummation of fiber.** The daily recommendation for women is 28–31 grams of fiber per day, and for men, it's 28–34 grams a day. Some great sources of fiber are flaxseed, lentils, and leafy green vegetables.

11. **Make your last meal of the day protein only.** A protein shake is a good final meal, and half a scoop of protein before bed can help your body avoid metabolising any muscle while you sleep.

12. **Where possible, eat organic fruits, vegetables, and grains and humanely raised, organic meats that are free of pesticides, hormones, antibiotics, and preservatives.** The more natural the better!

13. Optional: drink 1–2 cups of naturally caffeinated beverages per day. This could include black coffee, if coffee meshes well with your body, with no sweeteners and ideally no dairy. If coffee is not an option, you can also drink green tea, which studies have shown can help burn calories at rest, or any other herbal tea or black tea. Some studies say drinking caffeine can be very beneficial to overall health and weight loss. I invite you to conduct some further research.

14. Drink water with lemon (lemon optional) all day and ensure you are drinking at least 8-10 cups of water per day. Monitor your hydration levels (learn more about the importance of hydration in Appendix B)] and carry your water bottle with you religiously wherever you go. Where possible, drink from glass, not plastic. Plastic leaches chemicals linked to conditions such as estrogen dominance and other hormonal imbalances. Filtered water is ideal as this will aid in healthy liver functioning, cleansing of the system and will support your metabolism. I drink 2-3 liters of water a day.

15. Listen to your body. If something does not sit right with you after eating, substitute it for something that does. Bloating, fatigue, mental confusion, depression, anxiety, constipation, diarrhea, and cramps are all great examples of signs that a food is not sitting well with your particular body type. Be sure to journal your physical, emotional, and mental responses, and omit foods that don't work for you. If you`re unsure, get an allergy or food intolerance test.

16. When out of the house or traveling, carry a cooler bag with any meals you will need while you're out. Remember to pack some healthy snacks so you don't need to dash through a drive-through restaurant or munch on a chocolate bar when hunger pangs arise. However, if you eat according to these guidelines, you should notice hunger cravings diminish, if not disappear altogether. Healthy snacks include a handful of nuts (like almonds) with a piece of fruit (like an apple), organic boiled eggs, or smaller portions of a previous meal.

Here are some additional tips to help you stick to your guidelines while traveling: Before leaving on a jet plane, eat a good meal to get through the travel period. A healthy breakfast of oatmeal or a slow-acting carb like an apple is best! An oatmeal breakfast will leave you feeling satiated enough to get you through the airport without the need to hit up the fast-food chains on your way to the terminal. Purchase unsalted nuts, ready-to-go vegetables and fruits for the trip, and pack a cooler bag in your luggage with fruits, veggies, nuts, tuna pouches, or lean organic sandwich meats for when you arrive at your destination. Obviously, you will have to take into account what types of foods you are allowed to transport before packing your cooler bag.

Come prepared with your grocery list—you can get local produce when you arrive at your destination and prepare your food for day trips, which will help you avoid fancy buffets with rich foods. To avoid overindulging, keep to one treat meal every week. You will still feel like you are on vacation without all the extra calories. While I'm not a huge fan of protein bars (most are full of sugary junk), in emergencies a good quality protein bar (with as little sugar as possible) is better than chocolate or fast food. Carry your water bottle everywhere, and make sure you are sipping water throughout the day. If you choose to drink alcohol while on vacation, alternate between an alcoholic beverage and a bottle of water. Choose alcoholic drinks with little to no sugar where possible. Bring your journal with you wherever you go, revisit your goals daily, and remember why you are doing all of this. When eating out, choose wisely from the menu. Stick to lean proteins and vegetables, like organic chicken breast and asparagus. Ditch the sugary dessert, bread baskets, and request all sauces and dressings on the side. If you like hot sauce like I do, carry a small-size hot sauce in your purse or small baggie of dried chili flakes.

Walk to as many destinations as possible, instead of taking cabs or buses. If you like to go on cruises, do what some of my clients do and hire a personal trainer on the ship for two to three sessions. This can be enormously helpful in keeping you motivated and on track while vacationing. Check with your accommodations to see if there are amenities such as a fridge, toaster oven, or kitchenette. Stay in accommodations that have their own gym so you can squeeze in a quick workout before your day starts. If your accommodations don't have a gym, I highly recommend purchasing an exercise band to take on your travels. It's a low-cost, versatile, small piece of equipment you can use anywhere, any time, and can be used to train your entire body. I carry a band with me everywhere I go, and I also have one in my car.

17. Treats! Once a week, indulge in healthy treats. Note the word *healthy* and the word "treat" not "cheat," which can evoke limiting emotions or beliefs like "I did something wrong. I cheated." A bag of candy is not considered a healthy treat. A meal out at a restaurant is, or perhaps a glass of red wine. You still need to enjoy your life, and no great damage will be caused by munching on a healthy treat every now and again.

All you need is love. But a little chocolate now and then doesn't hurt.

Charles M. Schulz

At this point in my life, my favorite treat foods are chocolate, chicken burgers, and coffee. In the past, I also used to enjoy creamy pastas and frozen yogurt. I still do once in a while.

It's not easy to change what we eat. But we do the best we can.

So yes, you can eat an ice cream, but only every now and again. These are not to be considered weekly treats, but rather "on occasion" treats. Also, a treat is not a treat when you are having more than two a week! Eating more than two treats a week will start having a negative effect on your health, impeding your ability to transform your body and to lose unhealthy fat. Plus it can sabotage your attempts to take on new habits. Your body will need a certain period of abstinence to effectively adapt. Reintroduce treats—every now and then—after you have made progress on your weight-loss goals, and when you know you have developed enough inner strength not to use a treat to go off the rails. I suggest limiting your treats to once or twice a week.

Overall, follow the 80/20 rule: eat healthy and clean 80 percent of the time. Some clients I know save their treats until the weekend. However, I caution you to not radically change your eating behaviors from the week to the weekend, as this can lead to an unhealthy habit of binge eating.

Nowadays there are heaps of healthy ways to treat yourself. I encourage you to seek out healthy treat recipes that taste just as good as your favorite chocolate bar or ice cream, or buy yourself a healthy cookbook with recipes you will enjoy.

And those are the guidelines. Too easy! To put all of the recommendations into practice, try the following twelve-week sample meal plan from registered holistic nutritionist Kristina Graham. Note: The meal plan provided is a sample meal plan only. You should always consult with your physician, treating medical practitioner, or registered dietician to discuss the appropriate daily calories and macronutrient ratios for your specific needs as well as have a dietician or nutritionist review these guidelines to ensure they can be customized for you. Everyone has a unique body chemistry, different goals, and any set nutrition plan should be customized for every individual.

WEEK ONE	MONDAY	TUESDAY	WEDNESDAY	THURSDAY	FRIDAY	SATURDAY	SUNDAY
	Warm water with juice from ½ freshly squeezed lemon	Warm water with juice from ½ freshly squeezed lemon	Warm water with juice from ½ freshly squeezed lemon	Warm water with juice from ½ freshly squeezed lemon	Warm water with juice from ½ freshly squeezed lemon	Warm water with juice from ½ freshly squeezed lemon	Warm water with juice from ½ freshly squeezed lemon
Meal #1	4 egg-white (organic, free range) omelette with 2 tbsp diced onion, 2 tbsp diced red pepper, 1 tsp garlic, and ¼ cup cooked chopped chicken, sautéed in 1 tsp coconut oil. Serve with 1 slice of sprouted whole grain bread and a slice of tomato 1 cup blueberries	Protein shake with 1 cup raw spinach, 2 cups chopped kale, 1 cup blackberries, and 1 tbsp ground flaxseed	½ cup cooked steel-cut oats with ¼ cup unsweetened almond milk 4 egg whites scrambled 1 medium pear	4 egg whites scrambled with 1 tsp fresh parsley, 2 tbsp chopped green onion, and 1 tbsp sun-dried tomatoes 1 sprouted whole grain English muffin 1 cup raspberries	Protein shake with 1 cup raw kale and 1 cup blackberries	1 cup plain Greek yogurt with 1 cup raw pomegranates 2/3 cup cooked quinoa flakes with ¼ unsweetened almond milk	Protein shake 1 cup swiss chard 1 cup fresh strawberries
Meal #2	Protein shake 1 medium nectarine	½ cup plain Greek yogurt with 1 cup pomegranate seeds and 1 tbsp raw sunflower seeds 3 celery sticks	Protein shake 1 medium peach	Protein shake 1 pear	4 egg whites scrambled with 1 cup raw spinach 1 medium apple	Protein shake 1 nectarine	½ can water-packed tuna on top of 2 brown rice cakes 1 pear
Meal #3	4 oz grilled chicken breast on top of 3 cups of baby spinach, 2 oz alfalfa sprouts, ½ cup cooked black beans, 1 cup cucumber slices, ½ cup cooked quinoa with 1 tsp flaxseed oil	Pasta salad with 1 can tuna packed in water, 1 cup cooked brown rice penne, 1 cup sugar snap peas, ½ cup sliced radishes, and 1 tbsp of fresh chopped cilantro with 1 tsp olive oil and fresh lemon juice	4 oz baked tilapia with 1 cup baked sweet potatoes Salad made of 2 cups shredded cabbage with ½ cup roasted beets, 1 tbsp raw pumpkin seeds, and 1 tsp flaxseed oil	1 can of water-packed tuna on top of 2 cups raw spinach with 2 tbsp goji berries, ¾ cup cooked quinoa, and 1 tsp flax seed oil	4 oz grilled chicken breast on top of 1 cup quinoa fusilli pasta, with ½ cup tomato and basil pasta sauce, 1 cup grilled zucchini, and 3 sauteed baby bok choy	4 oz baked tilapia on top of 3 cups raw spinach with 1 cup roasted beets, ½ cup cooked kidney beans, and 1 tsp olive oil	5 oz grilled wild salmon on top of 2 cups dandelion greens with ¼ cup shredded carrot, 1 tbsp apple cider vinegar, and 1 tsp flaxseed oil, joined by 1 cup baked sweet potato

Meal #4	½ can of tuna packed in water, 1 cup baby carrots, and 1 cup raw zucchini slices with 2 tbsp hummus	1 cup red pepper slices with 4 tbsp black bean dip 10 raw almonds	4 oz grilled chicken breast with 2 tbsp hummus 1 cup raw sugar snap peas	1 cup raw cauliflower 1 cup raw broccoli 10 raw almonds	2 brown rice cakes with 1 tbsp natural almond butter 1 can water-packed tuna	2 oz grilled chicken breast with 2/5th of an avocado and 3 celery sticks with 1 tbsp sunflower seed butter	2 tbsp black bean dip with 1 cup raw cauliflower and 1 cup sugar snap peas
Meal #5	4 oz baked cod topped with 2 tbsp mint chutney along with 1 cup roasted spaghetti squash, 1 cup steamed baby bok choy, and 1 cup steamed asparagus	4.5 oz cooked boneless, skinless turkey breast along with 1 cup steamed broccoli, 1 cup steamed cauliflower, and 1 cup steamed carrots	4 oz baked, boneless, skinless chicken breast 3 cups mixed leafy greens with shredded carrots, celery, green onions, red onions, and grape tomatoes with 1 tsp olive oil	4 oz baked wild salmon on top of 3 cups of mixed leafy greens with shredded carrots, celery, green onions, red onions, and grape tomatoes with 1 tsp olive oil	5 oz baked turkey breast with 1 cup steamed asparagus and 1 cup steamed brussels sprouts	4.5 oz cooked shrimp on top of 3 cups of mixed leafy greens, 1 cup mushrooms, 1 cup chopped zucchini, shredded carrots, celery, green onions, red onions, and grape tomatoes with 1 tsp olive oil	4.5oz grilled turkey breast topped with 2 tbsp salsa with 2 cups chopped cabbage and 1 cup steamed asparagus
CALORIES (kCal)	1452	1425	1425	1459	1440	1425	1426
PROTEIN (grams)	147 g	147 g	145 g	142 g	144 g	146 g	146 g
CARBS (grams)	158 g	158 g	164 g	150 g	162 g	158 g	165 g
FAT (grams)	28 g	27 g	28 g	30 g	26 g	28 g	20 g

WEEK TWO	MONDAY	WEDNESDAY	THURSDAY	FRIDAY	SATURDAY	SUNDAY
	Warm water with 1 tbsp apple cider vinegar	Warm water with 1 tbsp apple cider vinegar	Warm water with 1 tbsp apple cider vinegar	Warm water with 1 tbsp apple cider vinegar	Warm water with 1 tbsp apple cider vinegar	Warm water with 1 tbsp apple cider vinegar
Meal #1	4 egg whites scrambled with 1 tbsp green onion, 2 tbsp diced red pepper, sautéed in 1 tsp of coconut oil with ¼ cup chopped cooked chicken; Sprouted whole grain English muffin; 1 cup pineapple	Protein shake with 1 cup swiss chard and 1 cup blackberries	4 scrambled egg whites on top of 2 slices spelt bread and 1 slice of tomato; 1 cup strawberries	1 cup plain Greek yogurt with ¼ granola and 1 cup blueberries	1 cup cooked quinoa with 1 tbsp cinnamon, 1 tbsp sliced almonds, 1 cup raspberries, and ¼ cup unsweetened almond milk; 4 egg whites scrambled	Protein shake with 1 cup chopped kale and 1 pear
Meal #2	Protein shake; 1 cup cherries; 1 cup raw spinach	¾ cup plain Greek yogurt with 1 cup blueberries; ¼ cup cooked steel-cut oats with 1 tsp cinnamon, 1 tbsp sliced almonds, and 1 tbsp ground flaxseed	Protein shake with 1 cup chopped kale and 1 cup mango	Protein shake with 1 cup chopped kale and 1 medium peach	Protein shake; 1 medium apple	4 egg whites scrambled with 1 tbsp diced onion, ¼ cup chopped peppers sautéed in 1 tsp coconut oil, with 1 slice of kamut bread
Meal #3	4 oz baked cod with 1 cup arugula, 1 cup dandelion greens, ½ cup cooked quinoa, 1 cup steamed green beans, 1 tsp olive oil, and ½ squeezed lemon	4 oz cooked ground turkey with 1 cup cooked elbow quinoa pasta, ½ cup of tomato and herb pasta sauce, 1 cup grilled mushrooms, and 1 cup grilled zucchini	4 oz grilled chicken breast on top of 2 cups swiss chard with ½ cup cooked lentils, 1 cup raw broccoli, and 1 cup raw cauliflower	5 oz baked chicken breast on top of 3 cups mixed field greens with 1 tbsp sesame seeds, 2 tbsp alfalfa sprouts, and 2 tbsp avocado oil, with 1 cup roasted sweet potatoes	4 oz grilled chicken breast on top of 4 cups raw spinach with ½ cup cauliflower, ½ cup broccoli, 1 tbsp apple cider vinegar, and 1 tsp flaxseed oil	Pasta salad with 1 can water-packed tuna, 1 cup cooked brown rice macaroni, 1 cup green beans, ½ cup chopped cucumber, 1 stalk celery chopped, and 1 tsp olive oil

Meal #4	½ *can water*-packed tuna with 1 cup chopped celery, 1 cup grape tomatoes, and 1 cup sliced green peppers	1 can water-packed tuna with 1 cup mixed field greens and 1 tbsp raw pumpkin seeds	½ *can of water*-packed tuna with 1 cup sliced cucumber and ¼ cup alfalfa sprouts	1 cup raw carrots and 2 celery sticks with 4 tbsp hummus	½ *can water*-packed tuna and ¼ cup chopped cucumber wrapped in a sprouted whole-grain tortilla	1.5 oz cooked shrimp with 2 tbsp shrimp cocktail sauce and 1 cup raw broccoli
Meal #5	4 oz baked chicken breast with 1 cup steamed baby bok choy, 1 cup steamed brussels sprouts, and 1 cup steamed carrots	4 oz baked tilapia with 1 cup roasted spaghetti squash and 1 cup steamed baby bok choy	4 oz baked salmon with 1 cup zucchini, 1 cup mushrooms, 1 cup red pepper, and 1 clove of garlic sautéed in 1 tsp coconut oil	4.5 oz grilled turkey breast topped with 2 tbsp salsa, along with 1 cup steamed green beans and 1 cup steamed broccoli	4 oz wild tuna steak with 1 cup kale, 1 cup mushrooms, 1 cup zucchini, ½ cup red peppers, and 1 clove of garlic sautéed in 1 tsp coconut oil	4 oz grilled chicken breast on top of 4 cups of mixed leafy greens with shredded carrots, celery, green onions, red onions, and grape tomatoes with 1 tsp olive oil
CALORIES (kCal)	1452	1434	1431	1452	1430	1426
PROTEIN (grams)	146 g	142 g	147 g	140 g	142 g	149 g
CARBS (grams)	160 g	166 g	155 g	168 g	160 g	165 g
FAT (grams)	27 g	26 g	29 g	29 g	28 g	21 g

WEEK THREE	MONDAY	TUESDAY	WEDNESDAY	THURSDAY	FRIDAY	SATURDAY	SUNDAY
	Warm water with juice from ½ freshly squeezed lemon	Warm water with juice from ½ freshly squeezed lemon	Warm water with juice from ½ freshly squeezed lemon	Warm water with juice from ½ freshly squeezed lemon	Warm water with juice from ½ freshly squeezed lemon	Warm water with juice from ½ freshly squeezed lemon	Warm water with juice from ½ freshly squeezed lemon
Meal #1	4 egg whites scrambled with 1 tbsp green onion, 1 cup spinach, 2 tbsp red pepper, ¼ cup chopped cooked chicken, sautéed in 1 tsp coconut oil. Served with one tomato slice and 1 slice sprouted whole-grain toast. 1 cup blackberries	¾ cup plain Greek yogurt 1 sprouted whole-grain English muffin with 1 tbsp natural almond butter 1 pear	Protein shake with 1 cup raw spinach and 1 cup strawberries	1 cup puffed brown rice cereal with ¼ cup unsweetened almond milk 1 cup plain Greek yogurt with 1 cup blueberries	4 egg whites scrambled with 1 cup spinach, 1 tbsp green onion, 2 tbsp red pepper, and ¼ cup chopped cooked chicken. Serve with 1 slice sprouted whole grain toast and 1 tomato slice. 1 apple	Protein shake with 1 cup swiss chard and 1 cup raspberries	4 egg whites scrambled with 1 cup spinach and 1 tbsp green onion, served with 2 slices of spelt toast and a slice of tomato 1 cup blackberries
Meal #2	Protein shake with 1 cup raw spinach and 1 medium apple	Protein shake	4 egg whites scrambled with 1 cup chopped red pepper wrapped in a sprouted whole-grain wrap 1 peach	Protein shake with 1 cup chopped kale and 1 pear	Protein shake with 1 cup spinach and 1 cup pomegranate seeds	¼ cup chopped cooked chicken with 2 tbsp hummus and 3 celery sticks 1 pear	Protein shake with 1 cup chopped kale and 1 nectarine
Meal #3	4.5 oz baked turkey breast with 1 cup cooked quinoa, 1 cup steamed kale, and 1 cup steamed carrots	4 oz boneless chicken breast on top of 3 cups of dandelion greens with ½ cup chickpeas, ½ cup cucumber slices, 1 tsp olive oil, and a squeeze of fresh lemon	4 oz lean ground turkey with 1 cup cooked quinoa pasta, ½ cup tomato with garlic pasta sauce, 1 cup zucchini, ½ cup chopped onion, and 1 clove of garlic 2 cups of mixed greens with 1 tsp flax seed oil	4 oz boneless chicken breast on top of 3 cups of shredded romaine lettuce, ½ cup cucumber, ½ cup roasted sweet potato, 1 tsp olive oil, and a squeeze of fresh lemon juice	4 oz baked wild salmon with ½ cup brown rice, 1 cup steamed bok choy, and 1 cup steamed green snap beans	4 oz boneless chicken breast with 1 cup cooked quinoa, 4 cups of raw spinach, ¾ cup shredded carrots, 1 cup green snap beans, 1 tsp olive oil, and a squeeze of lemon	4 oz baked trout with 1 cup cooked quinoa pasta, ½ cup steamed cauliflower, 1 cup steamed broccoli, and 1 tsp olive oil

Meal #4	½ cup water-packed tuna mixed with ¼ of an avocado on top of 2 brown rice cakes	½ cup cooked chopped chicken and 2 tbsp of hummus wrapped in two large lettuce leaves	½ can water-packed tuna with ½ cup chopped cucumber	½ cup chopped chicken breast with 1/5 of an avocado and 10 brown rice crackers	1 cup plain almond yogurt ½ can water-packed tuna	1 can boneless wild salmon with 1 cup lettuce and ½ cup chopped cucumber, wrapped in two small sprouted whole-grain wraps	½ cup plain Greek yogurt with 1 tbsp pumpkin seeds 3 celery sticks with 2 tbsp black bean dip
Meal #5	4 oz baked cod with 1 ½ cups steamed asparagus and 1 cup steamed bok choy, with a squeeze of fresh lemon juice	4 oz baked wild salmon with 1 cup roasted spaghetti squash and 1 cup steamed brussels sprouts	5 oz boneless chicken breast with 1 cup steamed broccoli, 1 cup steamed cauliflower, and ½ cup steamed carrots	5 oz baked cod topped with 2 tbsp mango chutney, along with 1 cup mushrooms, 1 cup asparagus, 1 cup red pepper, and 1 garlic clove sautéed in 1 tsp of coconut oil	4 oz baked turkey breast on top of 1 cup chopped kale, 1 cup chopped red cabbage, ½ cup shredded carrots, 1 tbsp sunflower seeds, and 1 tsp grapeseed oil	4 oz baked haddock with 1 cup sautéed rapini, 1 cup mushrooms, and 1 yellow pepper	5 oz baked chicken breast on top of 2 cups of mixed leafy greens with shredded carrots, celery, green onions, red onions, and grape tomatoes, with 1 tsp of flaxseed oil
CALORIES (kCal)	1453	1453	1467	1427	1438	1446	1426
PROTEIN (grams)	142 g	146 g	141 g	147 g	143 g	145 g	145 g
CARBS (grams)	165 g	158 g	161 g	158 g	158 g	162 g	164 g
FAT (grams)	30 g	30 g	29 g	27 g	29 g	24 g	26 g

WEEK FOUR	MONDAY	TUESDAY	WEDNESDAY	THURSDAY	FRIDAY	SATURDAY	SUNDAY
	Warm water with 1 tbsp apple cider vinegar	Warm water with 1 tbsp apple cider vinegar	Warm water with 1 tbsp apple cider vinegar	Warm water with 1 tbsp apple cider vinegar	Warm water with 1 tbsp apple cider vinegar	Warm water with 1 tbsp apple cider vinegar	Warm water with 1 tbsp apple cider vinegar
Meal #1	3 oz baked spinach with 1 cup of raw spinach wrapped in a sprouted whole-grain tortilla 1 orange	4 egg whites scrambled with 1 tbsp green onion and 2 tbsp red pepper, along with 1 slice of sprouted whole-grain toast and a slice of tomato 1 cup cherries	Protein shake with 1 cup chopped kale and ¾ cup of pomegranate seeds	1 cup plain Greek yogurt with 1 tbsp cinnamon, ¼ cup granola, and 1 cup blackberries	4 egg whites scrambled with 1 tbsp green onion, 2 tbsp red pepper, and ½ cup chopped kale with ½ sprouted whole-grain English muffin 1 cup blueberries	Protein shake with 1 cup chopped kale and 1 cup raspberries	4 egg whites scrambled with 1 cup chopped spinach, 1 tbsp green onion, and 2 tbsp red pepper, with 1 slice sprouted whole-grain toast and 1 slice of tomato 1 cup strawberries
Meal #2	Protein shake with 1 cup chopped kale 1 nectarine	Protein shake with 1 cup spinach and 1 cup strawberries	4 egg whites scrambled with 1 cup spinach wrapped in a sprouted whole-grain tortilla 1 cup blueberries	Protein shake with 1 cup chopped kale and 1 pear	Protein shake with 1 cup spinach and 1 apple	1 cup plain Greek yogurt with 1 cup pomegranate seeds and 1 tbsp sliced almonds	Protein shake with 1 cup raw kale and 1 medium peach
Meal #3	Taco salad with 4 oz grilled boneless chicken breast on top of 4 cups of raw spinach, with ½ cup cooked quinoa, ½ cup black beans, and 2 tbsp salsa	1 can of water-packed tuna with 1 cup cooked buckwheat pasta, 1/5 of an avocado, 2 tbsp alfalfa sprouts, ½ cup chopped cucumber, 1 cup chopped kale, and 1 cup chopped sweet peppers	4 oz baked boneless chicken with ½ cup cooked brown rice, 1 cup steamed green beans, and 1 cup steamed zucchini	4 oz baked cod with ½ cup cooked quinoa, ½ cup chopped cucumber, and ½ cup cauliflower *on top of 3 cups of dandelion greens with 1 tsp flaxseed oil*	4 oz cooked lean ground turkey with 1 cup brown rice pasta, ½ cup tomato and basil pasta sauce, 1 cup zucchini, 1 cup mushrooms, ½ cup onion, and 1 garlic clove sautéed in 1 tsp coconut oil	4 oz boneless chicken breast with 1 cup baked sweet potato topped with 1 tbsp chopped walnuts and 1 tbsp pure maple syrup, along with 1 cup steamed kale	4 oz cooked shrimp on top of 3 cups of dandelion greens with 1 cup chickpeas, 1 cup chopped cucumber, and 1 tsp olive oil

Meal #4	2 oz baked chicken with ½ cup chopped cucumbers and 3 celery sticks	1 cup raw broccoli, 1 cup raw cauliflower, and 1 tbsp pumpkin seeds with 2 tbsp hummus	½ cup water-packed tuna wrapped in 2 large lettuce leaves	1 cup shredded lettuce with 2 chopped hard-boiled eggs and 1 tbsp sprouted sunflower seeds	½ can water-packed tuna and 1/5 of an avocado wrapped in two large lettuce leaves	4 oz grilled chicken breast with 1 cup raw sugar snap peas and ½ sliced red pepper	2 oz grilled chicken breast with 1 cup roasted red beets topped with 1 tbsp chopped pecans
Meal #5	4 oz baked tilapia with 1 cup mushrooms, 1 cup shredded bok choy, 1 cup zucchini, 1 cup red peppers, and 1 garlic clove sautéed in 1 tsp of coconut oil	4 oz grilled salmon with 1 cup steamed asparagus, ½ cup steamed carrots, and 1 cup roasted red beets	4.5 oz baked turkey breast on top of 3 cups of field greens, ½ cup cherry tomatoes, ¾ cup shredded carrots, and 1 cup chopped sweet peppers, with 1 tsp olive oil and 1 tbsp balsamic vinegar	4 oz baked boneless chicken breasts with 1 cup steamed brussels sprouts, 1 cup steamed carrots, and 1 ½ cup steamed collard greens	4 oz baked tilapia with 1 cup steamed broccoli, 1 cup steamed carrots, and 1 cup steamed cauliflower	4 oz Ahi tuna steak on top of 1 cup shredded cabbage, 2 cups field greens, 1 cup steamed asparagus, and 1 cup cherry tomatoes with 1 tsp grapeseed oil	4 oz boneless chicken breast with 1 cup mushrooms, 1 cup red peppers, 1 cup chopped bok choy, 1 cup zucchini, and 1 clove of garlic sautéed in 1 tsp coconut oil
CALORIES (kCal)	1470	1430	1426	1450	1457	1455	1434
PROTEIN (grams)	142 g	143 g	146 g	142 g	141 g	147 g	147 g
CARBS (grams)	158 g	158 g	162 g	162 g	164 g	161 g	165 g
FAT (grams)	30 g	31 g	26 g	30 g	24 g	22 g	22 g

Rather than follow a specific meal plan, you can also simply refer to the following charts as you make your daily food choices:

Eat These Foods

VEGETABLES (1–2 cups)	PROTEINS (3–4 oz)	GRAINS (1/2–1 cup)
Asparagus	Turkey	Raw oatmeal
Broccoli	Lean beef (limit to twice a week)	Whole wheat breads, such as Ezekiel (1 slice)
Bell peppers	Bison (limit to twice a week)	Quinoa
Brussels sprouts	Chicken	Whole grain pasta
Mushrooms	Eggs (5 egg whites, or 1–2 yellows)	Brown rice
Red onion	Greek yogurt	Buckwheat
Swiss chard	Natural butters	Millet
Spinach	Tuna (limit to twice a week)	Whole grain pita
Arugula	Tilapia (or any white fish)	Whole grain tortilla
Carrots	Salmon	Couscous
Watercress	Legumes	*If you have an allergy or intolerance to wheat,
Celery	Beans	don't eat wheat products.
Beets	Chickpeas	
Artichokes	Lentils	
Romaine		
Snow peas		
Kale	**FRUITS (1 per day)**	**HEALTHY FATS (serving sizes below)**
Sweet potato (1 small)	Apples	Almonds (handful)
Bok choy	Limes	Egg yolks (2)
Zucchini	Lemons	Avocado (1/2)
Yams (1 small)	Oranges	Cashews (handful)
Squash	Bananas	Flaxseed (1 tsp.)
Cauliflower	Blueberries	Udos Oil 359 (check with your doctor first)
Ginger	Raspberries	Nut butter (1 tsp)
Garlic	Melon	Salmon (3–4oz)
Tomatoes	Watermelon (with seeds)	Walnuts (handful)
Cucumber	Grapes	Olive oil (1 tsp)
Sprouts	Pomegranate	Pecans (handful)
Leeks	Pears	Coconut oil (1 tsp)
Radishes	Dragon fruit	
Mixed greens	Kiwis	

Avoid These Foods

White flour	Fruit juice
White bread	Sausages
White pasta	Salamis
White rice	Any cured meats
Soda pop (including diet which is *worse!*)	Pork (Pigs don't sweat, so they don't release toxins. Yuk!)
Crisps (chips)	Fruit bars
Ice cream	Sugar-loaded protein bars
All dairy (some Greek yogurt is okay)	Sugary cereals
Chocolate (1 piece dark chocolate per day, once weight	Muffins
goal is achieved)	Scones
Fast food	Sugary spreads like jam or Nutella
Alcohol	Flavored milks
Cookies	Roasted nuts
Pastries	Tofu
Cakes	Chocolate/yogurt covered pretzels
Pies	Jell-O puddings
Fries	Candy
Sugary coffees	*All* artificial sweeteners and white/refined/processed sugars.
Hamburgers	(When desired weight and fat percentage is achieved,
Anything with trans fats	it's okay to add some sugar to your diet if you must, but
Donuts	choose from Sucranat, agave, fruits, honey, or any natural
Whipping cream	organic sugar.)
Soy	

With whatever approach you use, I encourage you to buy a food journal at the start of your transformation journey, so you can log and track your food intake for a while to get a good sense of what you are consuming on a regular basis. Food journaling also helps you make modifications and tweaks where necessary. If you have a smart phone, explore the numerous apps available that can track food and workouts. After a few weeks you will learn and get used to what your meals should look like as well as healthy portions and then you won't need to be as diligent with writing everything down and tracking it on a daily basis. Having said that, to this day I still pay very close attention to my nutrition and will at times log down my meals and track what I'm eating.

For additional information about nutrition and what is best for your unique body, I highly recommend consulting a registered dietician or holistic nutritionist.

CHAPTER 11

TRANSFORMING YOUR BODY: THE WORKOUT

If it doesn't challenge you, it will not change you.

The last chapter discussed the real health risks of consuming high-calorie, low-nutritive foods. But when you couple the typical Western diet with a sedentary lifestyle, the results can be downright devastating. Not only will it stack unhealthy fat pounds on your beautiful body, but it can potentially result in a significantly shorter life span and a whole range of deadly diseases. Our typical, sedentary, indoor lifestyle doesn't allow us to use the calories we consume. Sitting all day, every day, decreases your body's ability to burn calories, because electrical activity in the leg muscles shuts down, causing the muscles to atrophy and making it that much harder to exercise when the opportunity presents itself.

Another potentially devastating health risk of sitting for too long, especially for those with weight issues, is that the enzymes that breakdown fat drop by 90 percent when seated without a break for four hours or more a day. But don't worry—this chapter will give you a step-by-step exercise plan to use all the wonderfully healthy calories you consume, and increase your energy in the process!

Torch Fat and Reshape Your Body in Only 20 Minutes!

As you probably already know, there are many ways to change your body composition through exercise. If you don't currently follow an exercise regime, the most important thing is to simply get started and get that exercise ball rolling.

At this point in your transformation process, the workout I invite you to do is a total-body workout that requires only 20 minutes per workout on non-consecutive days, 3-4 times a week, to transform your body and your health.

This workout requires minimal equipment that you can do at the gym or in the comfort of your home (so you have no excuses, here). It will allow you to burn fat both during and after the workout, improve your cardiovascular performance, boost metabolism, improve heart health, and tone and sculpt your body—while also waking up and building your muscles. (See the full list of benefits below.)

Your workout prescription is for a 4-week period only, at which time you will need to switch your workout in order to continue challenging your body and producing results.

This workout is a circuit workout, and while the number of different circuit workouts you could do is truly limitless, I have designed this workout with several thoughts and intentions in mind. The first is that I wanted to present you with a workout that I know you will be able to do—nothing too complex, easy to follow, very little need for modification. Because it requires very little equipment and only 20 minutes a day, it is absolutely possible for *anyone* to carve out time for it in their daily schedule. (If you can't find 20 minutes in your day to dedicate to your health, then your current lifestyle is in need of drastic assessment and change.) Second, I want you to learn from experience that you don't need to perform hours upon hours of exercise a day to produce great results. In fact, doing so can have an adverse reaction, possibly spiking your cortisol levels and other causing other unnecessary health issues I don't want you to have to experience. Finally, circuit training is a highly respected and proven method of training to improve conditioning and both create muscle and burn body fat.

Benefits of The Workout

Here is a list of benefits of performing a workout like this one:

- Provides great results without a lot of time or specialized equipment
- Improves your resting metabolic rate in just one hour a week (yes, just three 20—minute workouts!)
- Improves strength and endurance through the resistance components of the circuit
- Increases likelihood of making regular exercise a lifestyle
- Enhances the look of your muscles and body shape
- Provides the opportunity to further improve your health by allowing more time for other necessary health activities, such as mind-body, stretching, and flexibility activities, like yoga and meditation
- May help improve insulin resistance
- May help to improve muscle imbalances

Did you know that a pound of body fat burns approximately 2 calories a day, while a pound of skeletal muscle burns up to approximately 6 calories per day? It pays to train your fabulous muscles in addition to cardio exercise. What's great about circuit training is that it combines both.

A Word about Safety and Rest

It's important to recognize that not all exercise types suit all "bodies," so before embarking on any new exercise program, including the circuit training program in this book, you should speak with your doctor. Although I've never come across a scenario where exercise was discouraged as a form of healing, the type of exercise you engage in should be considered and evaluated properly to determine whether it is best for you.

To prevent injury and stay safe while performing this circuit training program, it's super important that you read through and fully understand it before performing each exercise within the circuit. I also highly recommend performing in front of a mirror to start, or with a friend, so you can monitor your form and technique during each exercise. Practicing correct technique cannot be overstated. An exercise done poorly can cause more harm than good. Always maintain a neutral spine, never arch or round the back, and avoid locking out your joints. You should always maintain soft knees and elbows. Never extend an exercise to the point of pain. Take your body to the edge of its comfort zone, yes, but never push to the point of pain. The "no pain, no gain" mantra is just plain ridiculous. We do want to feel our muscles being challenged, but we also want to be able to lift our coffee cups to our lips the next morning, am I right?

It's also important that you don't ever train the same muscle group two days in a row. Following this practice ensures that you will get the rest and recovery your body needs for your muscles to grow and repair, and it is why the workout in this book is organized across non-consecutive days.

While performing your circuit, it's also very important that you are adequately hydrated, and should you experience any light-headedness, dizziness, acute pain, chest pain, or tingling in the arms, you should stop immediately and evaluate your situation, and/or call 911.

To achieve maximum benefits, ideally I'd like you to avoid resting at all between each exercise in the circuit, as this will greatly improve your fat-burning capacity. You can rest for one to two minutes between each circuit. You have two options to consider for your rest periods between circuits. First, you can rest completely and do no further movement at all—just stand there. The other option, which I highly recommend, is to either march, jog, or do a few jumping jacks or high knees in place for your rest period, depending on your fitness level.

Warming Up and Cooling Down

To further support your health and safety and to avoid injury, it's absolutely crucial that you always warm up your muscles with a 5-10 minute warm-up consisting of dynamic movements that will pump the blood around the body, loosen up your joints, and increase body temperature. Examples of some dynamic warm-up activities are: jumping jacks, light jump rope, light to moderate walking or jogging on the treadmill, gentle side lunges, or marching on the spot and swinging your arms.

At the end of your exercise activity you should always cool down with a lower, less intense movement for 2–10 minutes, such as some gentle stretching. If we don't perform a cool-down, we can experience what is called *venous pooling*, which is the accumulation of blood pooling in the veins, which can cause a drop in blood pressure or make you feel dizzy or lightheaded. Should this occur, a quick remedy is to lie on the ground face up and elevate your legs. The feeling should subside in a few minutes.

To increase mindfulness and to encourage the body to re-establish a healthy balance and homeostasis for post-workout activity; I also encourage my clients to finish their workouts with 3 deep breaths with their eyes closed and a 1–2 minute closed-eye meditation, releasing all thought and focusing on the natural rhythm of their breath only. A few moments of gratitude can also provide a fantastic frame for the remainder of your day.

Breathing

When performing all circuit exercises, it is absolutely critical that you breathe throughout the entire movement of each exercise—never hold your breath. Exhale (breathe out) during the most strenuous part of the movement (e.g., during the curling phase of a biceps curl, or pressing up through the heels in a squat).

What Weight Should I Start with and When Should I Increase It?

Start with a light weight to begin until you have perfected the correct form; at that point you can quickly progress to heavier weights when you're ready.

To assess the best size weight for greatest improvement, the last 2-3 reps of your set should be a challenge—you want to feel some burn in your muscles.

This is when your muscles are working at their best and are doing what they are supposed to be doing. If you don't fatigue and exhaust your muscles during each set, your muscles simply won't strengthen and grow, and we don't want that. We want you to see physical changes and growth.

A Word on Cardio

Because this workout is a circuit workout, meaning it's a proven form of body conditioning that targets both muscle strength *and* endurance, you are essentially doing your cardio while doing this workout. You don't need to be performing five hours of cardio activity like running or pounding on the treadmill every day to see and feel results. However, if you have a lot of fat mass to lose, then it can be advantageous to add more cardiovascular training to your weekly training regime. If you want to add more cardio, then I recommend performing an additional 20–30 minutes of moderate intensity cardio on the days you are not performing the workout. I also recommend speaking with a certified personal training or fitness professional that can help craft a customized cardio and strength training program based on your specific needs, fitness level, and goals. Remember, the purpose of this transformation journey, and of everything shared with you in this book, is not to produce a quick-fix remedy but a habit of practices that can become a lifestyle. Embarking on a mission of 5 hours of cardio and exercise a day is just plain insane, unless you were truly capable of maintaining this routine as an ongoing lifestyle. Even if you were physically able, I would still hope you wouldn't, given the adverse effect it would have long term. Think "slow and steady wins the race," if you really want long-term sustainable results.

Exercising with Heart Issues, Injuries, or Disease, or While Taking Medication

If you have any medical issues, take medication, have shoulder or knee injuries (or any injuries, for that matter), check with your doctor or treating physician first before exercising. Show them the circuit workout and exercises within this book and have them modify where necessary. I want you to get amazing results, but your health and safety must always come first!

The Workout

You will get out of your workouts what you put you in.

The following workout is a simple, at-home, sample circuit you can use to get started immediately on your physical journey. For best results, I encourage you to meet with a certified personal trainer in your area to discuss your unique body type and your goals, and to craft a customized training program for you.

As mentioned, I encourage you to find whatever type of exercise you find most enjoyable and what will awaken and nourish your body, mind, and soul. However, as someone who knows the enormous value and benefits of weight and resistance training, I encourage you to add this to your regular exercise regime. You won't end up with gigantic muscles, but what you will end up with is a powerful, strong, and fit body that will support the healthy functioning of your metabolism, improve your health and confidence, and strengthen your beautiful body.

How to Do

Begin by reviewing each movement and perfecting your form in front of a mirror or with a friend who can give you feedback. You can also watch me performing this workout by visiting my website, www.MichelleArmstrong. com/transformbook.

To perform the workout: Execute the suggested number of reps per movement, then move immediately on to the next movement, without resting until you complete the entire circuit. Rest one to two minutes between circuits, and perform two to three times depending on your current level of fitness. Where movements call for alternating parts of the body, such as the Lunge and Curl, perform the numbers of reps noted on each side.

Then, if you're feeling extra confident and/or you want to take it up a notch, add a twenty- to thirty-second high-intensity movement immediately after each circuit and before you rest. Two examples of high-intensity movements are:

1) jump rope (my favorite) or 2) high knees (running as fast you can on the spot with high knees).

Beginners, I suggest starting out with two circuits and no high-intensity movements. Increase your circuits and reps, and add in the high-intensity movements as you progress. Take a rest when you need it, but always seek to push yourself just that little bit further, as you'll be surprised at how capable you really are and how much more you can apply yourself. Increase your weights when confident and able.

Time

Each circuit will take approximately five to seven minutes to perform, depending on your speed. At all times direct your attention to your breath and your form while training, and feed yourself positive and uplifting words of affirmation and encouragement. You could even imagine I am right there with you, with my Australian accent, saying things like, "You can do it! Keep going! You've got this! I believe in you! You are strong and powerful. You can do anything! You can and you will achieve your goals, you spectacular and amazing human being!"

Equipment You Will Need

A workout mat or thick towel, three or more sets of dumbbells (5, 8, and 10 lbs.; go heavier when you can manage), and your beautiful and incredible body.

And now it's time to go through each of the moves.

The Moves

1. Squat Curl Press

Stand tall with your feet shoulder width apart, dumbbell in each hand, palms facing in. Lower your body, hinging at the hips as if you were sitting back onto a chair, ensuring your knees do not go over toes. Keep your core tight and chest high as you lower toward the floor. Pause for a second, then push your body back up to standing position through the heels. Stand tall again and, bending at the elbows, press the weights over your shoulders while keeping your core engaged. Lower your weights back to the start position and repeat.

Reps: 15-20

Muscled Worked: Legs, Glutes, Arms, Shoulders

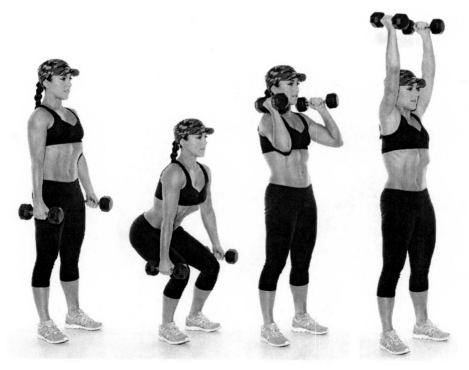

Squat Curl Press

2. Dumbbell Swing

Stand straight with your feet about shoulder-width apart, and hold the dumbbells with both hands in front of your hips. Push your hips back and then forward while maintaining a slight bend in the knee. The dumbbell will swing forward. Continue the motion of pushing your hips back and forward while swinging the weight. Keep your back flat during the entire motion and ensure all movement is being generated by the hips, as opposed to using your arms to swing the dumbbell. Avoid bending at the torso, and at the top of the movement squeeze and contract your glutes (your butt).

Reps: 15-20

Muscles Worked: Total Body

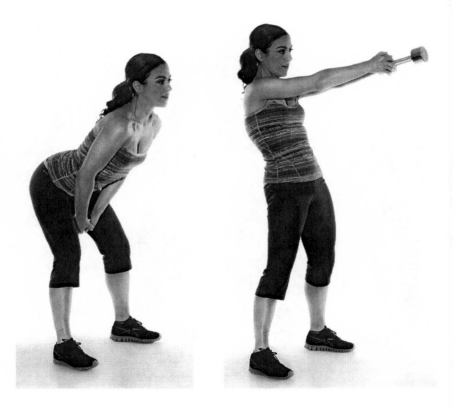

Dumbbell Swing

3. Lunge and Curl

Begin by standing upright, holding two dumbbells by your sides—wrists facing the body. Step forward with your left leg (a small step, not a big one), and lower your body, dropping your right knee to the ground. Ensure that your left knee does not travel beyond your toes as you come down, as this will put unnecessary stress on the knee joint. Now, using primarily the heel of your left foot, push up and back to the starting position. Once back to the starting position, keep your upper arms stationary and curl the dumbbells toward your shoulders. Hold briefly while you squeeze and contract your biceps, then slowly lower the dumbbells back to the starting position and repeat on the other leg. Keep your chest lifted high, and keep a neutral spine and engaged core.

Reps: 10-15 per side

Muscles Worked: Legs, Glutes, Arms, Shoulders, Core

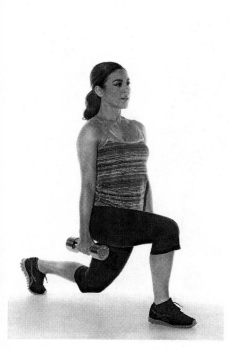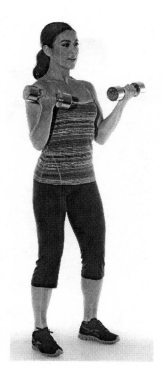

Lunge and Curl

4. Deadlift with Front Raise

Stand tall with your feet shoulder-width apart, your core engaged, and your chest high. Hold your weights in front of your thighs with your wrists facing your body. Your knees should be soft and not locked. Then, leading with your chest, bend at the hips while keeping your eyes forward (do not drop your head, as this will cause your back to round), and lower your torso as low to the ground as possible while maintaining a flat back. Pause for a second; then return to the start position, visualizing the back of your legs and your glutes pulling you upright.

Pause for a second, adjust your back to a normal stance, exhale, and raise your arms from the shoulders up no higher than shoulder height. Lower to the start position and repeat.

Reps: 12-15

Muscles Worked: Legs, Glutes, Back, Shoulders

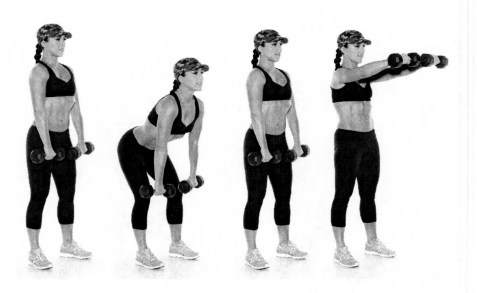

Deadlift with Front Raise

5. Plank Hops

Begin by positioning your body with your palms flat on the floor, fingers spread below your shoulders, with your knees bent up into your chest (as though you are in a crouched position). Then transfer the weight on to your palms, and while engaging your core, jump your feet back as far as you can into a plank position without letting your back dip toward the ground. Then immediately jump back to return to the starting position and repeat.

Reps: 12-20

Muscles Worked: Legs, Arms, Shoulders, Core

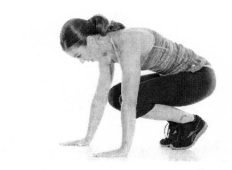

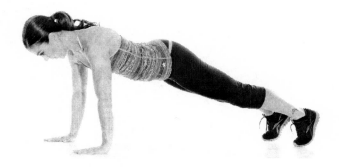

Plank Hops

6. Row with Rear Deltoids

Holding a dumbbell in each hand, soften your knees slightly and bend your torso forward, keeping your chest high and your head in line with your spine, ensuring you don't round your back. With your arms hanging towards the floor (wrists facing each other), engage your back muscles and pull your elbows up to your back, keeping them close to your torso. Squeeze your shoulder blades together for a slight pause and then return to the start position. Keeping your chest high and making sure not to round your back, raise your arms out to the side so your arms are perpendicular to your back. Return to starting position.

Reps: 12-15

Muscles Worked: Back, Shoulders

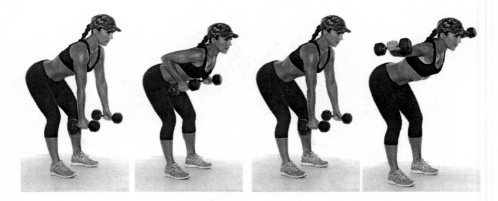

Row with Rear Deltoids

7. Side Raises

Stand tall, holding dumbbells by your sides, with palms facing your body. Without using your body to create momentum and with a slight bend in your elbow, tilt your hands slightly forward as though about to pour a glass of water, and raise your arms out to the side until they are parallel with the floor. Pause momentarily before lowering your arms back to the starting position.

Reps: 15-20

Muscles Worked: Shoulders

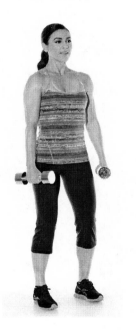 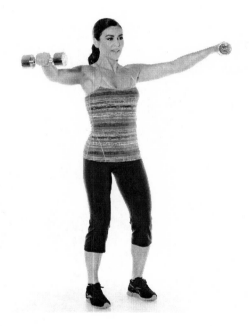

Side Raises

8. Chest Flys with Hip Raise

Lie on your back on a mat with your knees bent and close together, and draw in your heels toward your buttocks so that ideally you can touch your heels with your fingers. Your feet, knees, and hips should all be in line with each other. Hold a dumbbell in each hand by your chest, wrists facing the ceiling. Now raise your hips as high as you can (squeezing your glutes as you lift), and simultaneously bring your arms together so the weights are tracking over the nipple line. Arms should be straight, but your elbows should be soft and not locked. Then, holding your hips in this position for the entire movement, squeeze your glutes (your butt), and return your arms to the starting position.

(Suggestion: start with a light weight for this exercise until you master the form. The insertion point of the chest muscle being worked is small and can tear easily if the weight is too heavy and/or the correct form is not applied.)

Reps: 15-20

Muscles Worked: Chest, Butt, Legs

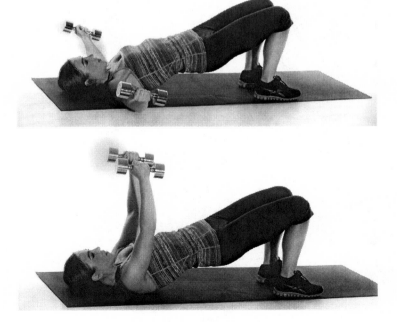

Chest Flys with Hip Raise

9. Superman

Lie face down on the floor and extend your arms out in front of you, thumbs up toward the ceiling. Then, using your lower back muscles, lift your chest along with your arms and your legs (which stay nice and straight) off the floor. Hold briefly before lowering your body back to the floor. Be sure your neck stays in line with your spine throughout the entire movement. Note: If you have any back problems, speak to your physician or back specialist before performing this movement or any of the movements within this circuit.

Reps: 12-15

Muscles Worked: Back

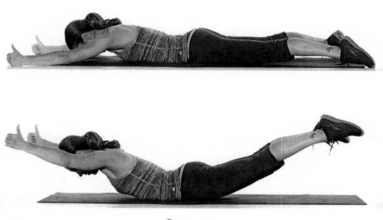

Superman

Tracking Progress

I encourage you to track your progress *every week*. Ongoing attention to your progress will help maintain adherence to the program and keep up your motivation as you see results—which, by the way, can come in many forms, and not just in physical appearance or a change in numbers of the scale. Despite belief to the contrary, your bathroom scale is *not* a good measurement or assessment of your progress. You can use the scale if you absolutely have to, but scales just measure total weight lost. A pound or more can be gained or lost due to stress, climate and elevation, water retention, hormonal fluctuations, and salt consumption. Plus, because muscle weighs more than fat, sometimes the scale can go up or stay the same even when you're actually losing body fat and getting healthier and leaner. So the assessment tools I want you to use are tape measurements; how you feel; improvements in strength, sleep, energy, and confidence; what you see when you look in the mirror; and how your clothes fit. To accurately assess your body composition, I recommend consulting with your doctor or an experienced personal trainer with access to professional body composition equipment or technology.

Mix It Up

After four weeks, it's important you switch up your workout, as our bodies adapt very quickly and we need to continually challenge our bodies with different exercises, routines, weights, and sets if we want to see noticeable changes.

The following tips are recommended to support you on your journey and ensure great results. You can choose one, some, or all. They are not mandatory—only ideas to assist you.

- Ask a friend or family member to train with you.
- Create a family or community health challenge and invite others to join you in your transformation toward a fitter body and better health.
- Blog about your experience and transformation online for accountability.
- Share your experience and transformation via Facebook for accountability.

- Create an Inspiration Board and cover it with inspiring quotes, words, images, mantras, and scriptures.
- Get at least 8 hours of sleep a night for adequate rest and recovery.
- Where possible, eliminate stressors in your life.
- Begin each workout with a meditation, setting your intentions for your session.
- End each workout with 3 deep breaths and a closing 1–2 minute meditation and gratitude session to center and focus your mind for your day.
- Write out your fitness goals and always have them in front of you while you train.
- Always eat a small meal before your workouts to provide your body with the energy it needs to exercise. Eat a small meal after your workout consisting of protein and a fast-acting carb to repair and nourish your muscles. A protein shake is a good choice.
- Take before and after photos for motivation and inspiration. Take one photo at the start, then one photo every week to track your progress.
- Take measurements to track your progress. Use a tape measure.
- Buy a workout journal and track your workouts.
- Start attending a weekly fitness class for inspiration and to mix up your cardio.
- Tell friends and family what you are doing and ask for their support and gentle encouragement on the days you may not feel like exercising.
- Email *me* your stories and experiences. I love hearing about other people's journeys, and although I receive tons of e-mails these days, I will do my best to get back to you.
- Pray and meditate each day for the support, strength, and courage to achieve your goals.
- Visualize your desired results.
- Post pictures, images, and post-it notes with inspiring messages around your home to keep you motivated and feeling positive.
- Buy yourself a healthy recipe book that falls in line with my Nutrition Guidelines.

- Get excited and motivated by the feeling of your muscles working during and after exercise. This is a sign of desired change. Avoid whining and moaning about the sensation. It's supposed to feel this way!
- After 4 weeks, investigate new ways to work out to avoid plateauing. Mix things up so you stay motivated by your workouts. Consult a personal trainer, go online and do an Internet search, buy some exercise DVDs, or join a local gym.
- Buy yourself a pedometer and track your steps on a daily basis. Your goal is 10,000 steps a day.

Contract to Self

This is an activity I have my clients perform at the beginning of their journey. It is a "Contract to Self"—a commitment to yourself to begin your journey of transformation and persevere regardless of what obstacles may arise. There will be times when you take two steps forward and one step back, and times when you fall off the exercise wagon altogether. This is normal, so expect it, but then get right back into the exercise saddle. Keep this contract with you at all times and post it in your training area for motivation and inspiration. Simply fill in the blanks on the contract, and then sign and date.

CONTRACT TO SELF

I, (insert your name), willingly choose to commit to making regular exercise and clean eating a lifestyle. I choose to embark on this journey because (insert 3–5 reasons), and although I foresee possible obstacles, such as (insert obstacles), arising at some point during my journey, I will not let them stop me from achieving my goals. Should I need assistance, support, or motivation at any time, I will call (insert 1–3 people who will lovingly encourage you and hold you accountable). When I find myself procrastinating or if I get stuck, I will tell myself the following 3 affirmations (insert 3 affirmations here). I promise that I will not give up on myself because I acknowledge that I deserve to have excellent health and a fantastic life, and because this journey of transformation is going to assist me in aligning with my calling and purpose in life. I will remind myself regularly that other people have experienced and are experiencing similar challenges, and if they can do it, I can too!

Signature: _____*Date:* _____

To succeed in your quest, you need to believe with every fiber of your being that you can do this—you can overcome any obstacle, and no matter what happens you will persevere and not give up. No matter the effort, you will do it and you will win! You will achieve the body and life you want. I believe in you. Believe in yourself and the power within you to succeed!

CONCLUSION: TIME TO FLY

The secret to your success is *you*. Nobody, including me, is going to tell you what to do or when to do it, and nobody is going to change your life for you. If you don't act, nothing will change. But if you do, *everything* will change. This is the essence of free will. You get to choose the quality of your life. You won't be punished or condemned if you don't act—life doesn't operate this way. But life will not swoop in and live your life for you. Instead it lovingly stands by, waiting for you to show up and tell it through your actions what you want. Then it swoops in to support you and give you everything you need.

You are quite entitled to toss this book aside and never think about it again. You can continue to sit on the sofa and daydream about your desires while eating yourself into a state of temporary bliss that moments later will dissolve into misery. You can remain inside your comfort zone and continue to avoid your feelings and fears. But is this *what you want?* Or did you pick up this book for a reason? Do you really want to repeat the past and continue to feel the way you feel? Or are you ready to experience all that life has to offer you—change, growth, transformation, and joy?

The power to transform yourself and your life lies within you. You just have to *believe* it. You get to decide. Life is so kind in this way. It doesn't force anyone to do anything they don't want to. Yet like a parent who loves her child, Life wants more than anything for *her* child to have an amazing life she loves and enjoys and to experience the best that life has to offer. Nobody is going to come over to your place and cram healthy food into your mouth or take you for a walk (unless perhaps you pay them, but even then it has to be your choice). Your life experience is your choice. You can choose to remain in an unhealthy and uncomfortable body and simply exist in an unfulfilling or meaningless life, *or* you can choose to experience a fabulous, joyful, and purpose-driven life that involves making yourself and your health a priority.

Action expresses priorities.

> *Gandhi*

Making ourselves a priority isn't selfish, because when we take care of ourselves first we have the power and capability to easily take care of others. Because so many of my clients long to make a difference in the world, to inspire others and help heal others through their innate sensitivity, empathy, and loving hearts, anything less than making themselves a priority isn't going to allow them to change the world, now—is it?

It's time to make yourself and your health a priority. You can no longer afford to put yourself last or even second on your list of priorities. You are going to have to start saying "no" to certain people in your life, certain distractions, and certain activities that do not support your goals and intentions. You are going to have to stop being a people pleaser and instead start listening to and acting on the voice inside your heart.

The whole purpose of life is to live your truth and unleash your passions into the world.

Life Is Calling You

We each have a calling in life. That calling is speaking to you now through the words in this book. It is inviting you to put an end to the abuse of your body and denial of your truth, and to start listening to the voice of your heart. You are here for a reason. What you do in this life matters. *You* matter, and it's time for you to know this. It's time to awaken to the essence of your soul—to start living the life you dream about in your head or are too afraid to dream about. Yes, this book is about weight loss, transforming your health, and living a more joyful life, but it's also about empowering you to awaken to your greatest potential. In all my years of practice, I have not met a single soul who, once healed from their pain and free of the behaviors that limited their lives, did not feel a calling to bring to this life something only they were capable of bringing. Life is nudging us gently all the time and whispering gentle and loving messages in our ears. We only need to stop and listen—to pay attention and be present to our physical, emotional, mental, and spiritual bodies, and we will *hear* what life is trying to tell us.

In short, life wants you to shine. It wants you to rise above your fears, achieve excellence, and live a life of passion, love, and joy. Life doesn't want you to suffer. It wants you to *live*.

Awaken to your calling. Remember who you are . . .

Everything that has happened to you happened with love and purpose—to guide you to your highest truth and reason for being. You are a gift to this world—a unique gift that only you can share with the world, because there is no other you anywhere else. You are a rare and exquisite gem, and you are here to radiate your beauty and truth with the world. Whether you are a plumber, teacher, electrician, accountant, realtor, doctor, musician, or bartender—the hat you wear is irrelevant—it's what you bring of *yourself* through your roles that adds value to this life and to the lives of others.

My purpose and my calling is to remind you of your magnificence, and to remind you how powerful and loved you are. My book is simply a vehicle to share this message, and I assure you that it's in your hands for a reason, and the reason is—*you are ready*. This is your time. This is your moment. Do not wait any longer to awaken to your magnificence and shine your light on to this world. The world needs *you*. It needs you to remember your essence and express your true self. You are being invited right now to let go of your past and all the stories associated with your past, and to embrace this moment and act out of what this moment is inviting you to do.

One day at a time and one step at a time is all it takes. Don't worry about all the other steps that you may need to take in the future, because you cannot control the future. Life is responsible for the future, and if you let it, it will take care of your future for you. You just need to focus on the present—*this moment now*.

I can think of no better way to conclude than to give you one final practice—the practice of gratitude. Gratitude can help to expand our awareness about what's happening in our lives, so we can see our experiences in new and uplifting ways.

I once worked with an amazing twenty-six-year-old woman named Janet, who had been paralyzed from the waist down since she was sixteen. Janet was in a wheelchair and had a degenerative condition that affects the neuromuscular system. Her condition was slowly robbing her entire body of movement, and she had no idea how long it would be before she became completely paralyzed. The truly inspiring thing about Janet was that she was able to experience gratitude for her situation. She said to me, "There's a reason I'm in this chair and I'm just going to make the most of it. If you think I'm bad off, you should see some of the friends I have—they can't even move their arms. I may not be able to walk, but I'm grateful I still have the use of my arms."

You can't and shouldn't compare your personal problems to someone else's, but that being said, other people's circumstances can provide an opportunity for you to develop an empowering perspective, to acknowledge to yourself just how much you do have in your life. The power of gratitude cannot be overstated. In gratitude, your whole sense of being shifts—your attitude, energy level, and perceptions change, and you feel lighter and brighter.

Practice: Gratitude

- For one week, every night before bedtime, write down all the things you are grateful for in your life. Keep this list with you during the day, so you can access it and add to it at any time. Acknowledge and express gratitude for all of the fabulous things in your life: a great family, a wonderful relationship, financial abundance, a lovely home, or an exciting career.

- If you feel you have nothing to be grateful for, focus on the things in your life you take for granted. Are you grateful for the fact that you can see, hear, breathe, or walk? Add those kinds of things to your list. Anything and everything is something to be grateful for.

- Your list should also include words of gratitude for yourself—for your dedication to your personal transformation, for your hard work, your commitment, your perseverance, your effort. Whether you lose 3 or 30 pounds in a month, acknowledge and affirm yourself through gratitude!

- Whenever you're stressed out, in a bad mood, and things aren't working in your life, or there're a lot of negativity going on, stop in the middle of what's happening, pull out your gratitude list and read it. Train your focus on the aspects of your life for which you are grateful.

- After a week, check in with yourself. How has practicing gratitude changed your attitudes, thoughts, and behaviors?

I encourage you to make the practice of gratitude a part of your daily life for the rest of your life. It is time to embark on a journey of faith. It's time to break out of the chrysalis and spread your wings and fly!

APPENDIX A: HORMONAL HEALTH

Throughout this book, we have discovered the incredible power our mindset can have over our physiology and life experiences. Yet it works both ways: our physiology also impacts and influences our mindset. Having a deeper understanding of the intimate relationship between our psychology and physiology will further empower and support you on your transformation journey. And one of the key physiological influences over our psychology is our hormones.

What Are Hormones?

So what are hormones, anyway—and why do you need to understand how they work? Hormones are chemicals produced by the endocrine system that get released into your body through the bloodstream and tissues. Put simply, hormones allow different parts of your body to communicate with each other. They impact your metabolism, immune system, energy level, sexual response, fertility, appetite, ability to cope with stress, emotional responses, and overall mood. The endocrine system is highly complex, so your hormone levels are affected by your age, gender, general health, diet, and genetic makeup, as well as by the amount of exercise and sleep you get. They are also affected by the time of day, month, and year.

When your hormones are in balance, you probably don't give them a second thought. But if something goes wrong, hormone imbalances can significantly impact your health, weight, and quality of life—producing symptoms that from a conventional medical perspective can look a lot like depression or an anxiety disorder.

For example, in my role as a stress coach and fitness trainer at the Institute of Hormonal Health in Ontario, Canada, I participate in the diagnostic process alongside the doctor and contribute to patients' holistic treatment plans for hormonal imbalance issues, such as adrenal fatigue, estrogen dominance, and thyroid issues. One common story I hear from the patients at the Institute for Hormonal Health, as well as from clients at my studio, goes something like this:

"I've done everything right. I am eating clean, I exercise regularly, and I meditate—but intuitively I just felt like something wasn't right inside. I finally went to the doctor, so the doctor could help me figure out what that 'something' was. But when I told her about my symptoms, she didn't run any tests or anything; she diagnosed me with depression on the spot, and prescribed an anti-depressant."

Most conventional medical doctors have not been trained to view emotional symptoms from a hormonal perspective. If you don't understand how your hormones work, and what symptoms typically indicate that they are out of balance, you could end up with mental health misdiagnoses and prescriptions for psychological medications that may numb the surface symptoms, but only exacerbate the true problem.

And that's exactly what happens for so many of our clients. After they receive a full round of testing at the Institute to determine their hormone levels, they often discover that they had been misdiagnosed—their symptoms were being caused by a hormonal imbalance, not depression. In other words, they had spent months or years on prescription medication they didn't need, loaded with side effects they never needed to endure in the first place! These stories break my heart, yet I hear them so often. The good news is that once patients are tested and receive the right support to bring their hormones back into balance, they heal relatively quickly and can't believe how great they feel!

So if you know you're doing "everything right" but still aren't experiencing the results you want, or if you just have that sense that "something isn't right inside," this appendix will provide you with some basic knowledge about 11 key hormones, to help you determine whether your hormones may be what's holding you back and what you can to do to get the support you need.

Estrogen and Progesterone

Estrogen and *progesterone* are the female sex hormones, and for optimal hormonal health, what's most important is that their ratio is a balanced one. Commonly known as the "belly fat hormone," estrogen is produced by the ovaries in increasing amounts throughout the duration of the menstrual cycle. Its partner progesterone is produced by the ovaries with ovulation and continues to be produced for the latter two weeks of the menstrual cycle.

Estrogen dominance is a term used to describe a relatively greater amount of estrogen relative to progesterone. This is typically seen in perimenopausal women who are no longer ovulating regularly. During the menstrual cycle, the amount of estrogen released is ideally balanced by the amount of progesterone released beginning at ovulation and throughout the rest of the cycle. But if one is not ovulating regularly, then progesterone is not being produced to any significant degree in the latter half of the cycle, resulting in too much estrogen relative to progesterone. Approximately 50 percent of women beyond the age of 35 are ovulating in only half of their cycles.

Estrogen dominance is also on the rise due the increasing amount of *xenoestrogens* we are taking into our body from the environment. Xenoestrogens are chemicals that mimic the actions of estrogen and can be found in the pesticides on food, plastic water bottles, drinking water, and more.

Symptoms of estrogen dominance include:

- Heavy periods
- Tender breasts/fibrocystic breast disease
- PMS
- Fibroids
- Endometriosis
- Frequent yeast infections

A woman is considered to have entered menopause once she has not had a menstrual period for more than one year. Physiologically, menopause is associated with a reduction in estrogen, as well as a significant reduction in progesterone. For many women, this decline in ovarian function and low levels of both estrogen and progesterone can be accompanied by a spectrum of symptoms in varying degrees of severity, including:

- Hot flashes
- Memory decline
- Anxiety
- Insomnia or sleep disruption
- Weight gain
- Decreased libido
- "Crawly" skin
- Frequent urinary tract infections
- Vaginal dryness with painful intercourse
- Frequent bladder infections
- Sleep disruption
- Low moods
- Osteopenia/osteoporosis

Testosterone

We may not often think of testosterone as part of our sex hormones, but women also produce testosterone in "surges" during their menstrual cycle, which contributes to libido. Our bodies produce testosterone from progesterone, which is also used to produce cortisol. If we are suffering from a cortisol imbalance or adrenal fatigue, our bodies will prioritize converting any available progesterone to cortisol first, to meet the demand of our stress response system (as whenever our stress response system is activated, our bodies believe we are in a life-or-death situation and are going to prioritize survival over sex!). Therefore adrenal fatigue can result in low levels of testosterone. Also, because the precursor to cortisol (and therefore to testosterone) is cholesterol, low-cholesterol diets can also contribute to low testosterone levels.

Symptoms of testosterone deficiency:

- Decreased sex drive
- Thinning of pubic and auxiliary hair
- Poor muscle recovery after a work-out
- Decreased muscle mass
- Osteoporosis/osteopenia

Thyroid (T3 and T4)

The thyroid gland is a butterfly-shaped structure at the base of the front of the neck. It is responsible for regulating metabolism throughout the body. Tri-iodothyronine (T3) and thyroxine (T4)—the hormones produced by the thyroid gland—are intimately interconnected with many other hormones. Disruption of your thyroid function can cause imbalances of other hormones; conversely, disruption of other hormones can cause thyroid imbalance.

Hypothyroidism—an under-functioning thyroid gland—is a very common condition affecting about 1 in 13 people. The symptoms of hypothyroidism are broad in range and may include depression, anxiety, weight gain, constipation, hair, skin, and nail changes, menstrual irregularities, cold intolerance, fatigue, and insomnia, to name but a few.

Currently, Canadian and American labs report a normal range for TSH (i.e., thyroid stimulating hormone—a blood marker for thyroid function) as 0.35-5.0 mIU/L, which is too broad a range according to the American Association of Clinical Endocrinologists, the National Academy of Clinical Biochemistry, and the American Academy of Anti-Aging Medicine. With a recommended reference range of 0.35-2.5mIU/L, fewer patients will have their symptoms of hypothyroidism and sub-clinical hypothyroidism overlooked. Treatment of hypothyroidism is helpful in balancing all hormones, as your thyroid plays such an integral role in optimal hormonal health.

An over-functioning thyroid, or *hyperthyroidism*, can also cause problems, including sudden weight loss coupled with increased appetite, rapid heartbeat, nervousness, anxiety, irritability, sweating, fatigue, muscle weakness, difficulty sleeping, thinning skin, fine, brittle hair, changes in menstrual patterns, increased sensitivity to heat, and other symptoms.[27] You have probably noticed that this list of symptoms overlaps quite a bit with the symptoms listed above from other hormonal imbalances – which underscores how difficult it is to self-diagnose hormonal imbalance and how important it is to get tested to discover where the true imbalance lies!

Cortisol

This hormone is deserving of more air time, as cortisol imbalance is frighteningly common. Our adrenal glands are pyramid-shaped glands that sit on top of each kidney, and play a role in producing multiple hormones, including progesterone, testosterone, estrogen, and cortisol. The role of cortisol is to help us manage all types of stress—emotional, physical (inflammation), and environmental. A long time ago, the stress response (also known as the "fight or flight" response) came in handy when we had to run to save our lives from wild animals, and fight off a nearby tribe from stealing our food. Today most of us experience this same fight or flight response while sitting in traffic, waiting in line at the bank, preparing for an interview or exam, making a presentation, or having a discussion about finances with a spouse.

So between cell phones and emails clamoring for our attention, fast-paced lifestyles, and environmental pollutants like pesticides and plastics taxing our hormonal systems, our adrenal glands are on overload. Because of this constant demand for cortisol production, there is a "steal" effect, whereby cortisol is produced in large amounts at the expense of other hormones. This can impact progesterone, estrogen, and testosterone production, causing an overall imbalance and hormonal dysregulation. In many cases, all of these hormones, including cortisol itself, cannot be maintained, and the result is burnout—otherwise known as cortisol dysregulation, or adrenal fatigue.

Upwards of 80 percent of North Americans suffer from some degree of adrenal fatigue, according to Dr. Kristy Prouse, founder of the Institute of Hormonal Health. Adrenal fatigue can disrupt not only estrogen, progesterone, and testosterone balance, but also thyroid function, brain neurotransmitter balance, and gastrointestinal function.

Adrenal fatigue, in all its mild and severe forms, is usually caused by some form of stress. Stress can be physical, emotional, psychological, infectious, or a combination of these. It is important to know that your adrenals respond to every kind of stress the same, whatever the source.
James L. Wilson, *Adrenal Fatigue: The 21ˢᵗ Century Stress Syndrome*

Some of the more common symptoms of adrenal fatigue include:

- Slow to wake up in the morning
- Ongoing fatigue throughout the day
- Craving for salt or salty foods
- Lethargy or lack of energy
- Increased effort to do everyday tasks
- Decreased sex drive
- Decreased ability to handle stress
- Increased recovery time from illness, injury, or trauma
- Lightheadedness when standing up quickly
- Mild depression
- Worsening PMS
- Foggy thinking
- Decreased tolerance of others
- Afternoon low at 3–4 pm
- Sleep disruption

Not surprisingly, cortisol dysregulation can also have a negative effect on our body composition. As Dr. Prouse points out, "When the body is experiencing prolonged levels of stress and releasing consistently high amounts of cortisol, it can play havoc on several other hormones such as estrogen and progesterone, which can cause weight gain or weight loss. It can also trigger unhealthy food habits such as cravings for sugary and salty foods, which also have a negative impact on our body and health. "To restore balance back to the body, it's crucial we learn how to reduce and manage stress in our lives and modify our diets by eliminating as much sugar as possible and eating more nutrient-dense foods. Exercise is also a powerful stress reliever and hormone balancer."

Other Hormones That Impact Weight

In addition to all of the hormones listed above, there are many other minor hormones that also impact hunger regulation and thus weight gain, such as melatonin (which regulates sleep), insulin (which regulates our blood sugar), leptin (known as the "obesity hormone"), ghrelin, neuropeptide Y (NPY), and cholecystokinin. Dysregulation of these hormones may be derivative from an imbalance in the other major hormones listed above, or simply by genetics. Clearly our hormonal balance plays a complex and integral role in our health and wellness!

So What if We Think We Have a Hormonal Imbalance?

If you think you may be experiencing a hormonal imbalance, here are five empowering steps you can take toward hormonal health:

Trust Yourself!

If deep down you feel something just isn't right, listen to what your intuition is telling you! For the vast majority of patients I've seen at the Institute, their instincts about their health were spot on. Medical professionals are wonderful people, and they are very smart. But they don't know everything, and they certainly won't know you better than you know yourself.

Get tested.

Visit a holistic medical practitioner who can organize a hormonal panel for you—make a list of all the symptoms you've noticed that are bothering you, and take the above hormone list to your first appointment as well.

Manage your stress.

Today people often refer to stress as "mental and emotional pressure." Whatever you call it, stress is an overwhelming feeling that can manifest emotionally and physically and reduces your ability to be present and productive or to remain calm and peaceful. Stress whips you out of your "centeredness" and, as we saw in the earlier section on cortisol imbalance, can have a very negative, if not deadly, impact on your life.

The clients I work with who have large amounts of stress in their lives find it much more difficult to manage their weight and achieve a healthy body composition than those who have little or no stress. Oftentimes I've had to work with a client on reducing the stressors in their life first before any physical changes in their body can be seen. Based on my experience, hormonal healing is more rapid in clients who not only address the chemical imbalance, but also change their diet, exercise, and embrace all the mind-body-spirit work we've already discussed in this book.

So in addition to all the practices we've already covered in Parts I, II, and III, here are some additional specific stress-relieving practices I recommend:

- Re-evaluate how your time is spent in relation to your life values
- Sleep at least eight hours a night
- Eliminate stressors in your life wherever possible, including toxic people and environments
- If unable to remove yourself from a stressful situation, learn to change your thinking about it
- Engage in laughter, which causes the body to relax (even if just briefly)
- Be assertive
- Avoid perfectionist behaviors

- Engage regularly in relaxing activities, such as yoga, meditation, and prayer, and practice relaxation techniques
- Learn how to respect your own time and say NO.

Do your own research.

Conduct your own research into the treatments being prescribed to you. Don't just accept what you're told. Now I'm not suggesting that you assume that what you're being told isn't accurate, because it might be. What I'm suggesting is that you take ownership of your health and your body because it is, after all, *your* body. If something doesn't feel right to you, be sure that you realize that you deserve the best possible care, and voice your feelings and concerns. If you don't feel your practitioner is listening to you, leave that practitioner immediately and go find someone who *will* listen to you. Mindful, compassionate, holistic practitioners are out there. You just may need to look a bit harder to find them.

Continue to listen to your body.

Even after your treatment begins, continue to listen to your body—physically, emotionally, spiritually, and mentally. Nearly every client I've worked with who has had a significant hormonal imbalance has also been experiencing a significant life test that has been challenging their abilities to cope. In that sense, view your hormonal imbalance and recovery process as a gift, in that it is giving you the opportunity to slow down and deeply re-evaluate your life and your current priorities. Keep your "awareness eyes" wide open so you can continue to learn and grow.

Summary

We are all up against significant saboteurs where our health and wellness and quality of life is concerned. Environmental toxins and pollutants. Nefarious manufacturing and production of our so-called food. Insanely fast-paced lifestyles. Lack of personal support and a sense of community. An outdated medical model that fails to see individuals as "whole persons" and instead relies on Band-Aid solutions in the form pharmaceutical interventions, which serve to line the back pockets of their manufacturers more than truly healing the individual's problem.

But this does not mean we are doomed. On the contrary, it just means we need to fight back. And how you do fight back? Through awareness, mindfulness practices, educating ourselves, developing your voice, sharing what you know with others, and taking personal responsibility for your health. As you do so, you will become an ambassador of hope, healing, and wellness for others.

You deserve to experience amazing health and a joyful, passionate, love-filled life. But if you want what is rightfully yours, you must be courageous and go out there and claim it!

APPENDIX B: NUTRITION BASICS

As we learned in chapter 10, it's hard to know what healthy eating even means anymore! So let's return to some nutrition basics.

Understanding Macronutrients

The main building blocks of nutrition are known as *macronutrients*, which include *carbohydrates*, *fats*, and *proteins*. The body needs large amounts of macronutrients to function at its best, and the best way to get all the macronutrients you need is to eat an organically grown, diverse, and balanced diet.

The Skinny on Carbohydrates

Carbohydrates supply the majority of the energy you need to stay alive on the most basic level and are vital to optimal health and performance. Unfortunately carbohydrates have developed a bad rap over the years, as people have come to believe that carbohydrates are fattening and unhealthy, which simply isn't true. Not all carbohydrates are created equal. Let me explain what I mean.

Complex carbohydrates are a necessary part of a healthy diet and keep the body functioning at an optimal level. You should not omit carbohydrates from your diet if you want a healthy, fit, and lean body. Some examples of complex carbohydrates include whole grains like quinoa, oats, millet, brown rice, and whole grain pasta, and legumes (which also provide protein) like black beans, lentils, and kidney beans. Whole-grain complex carbohydrates are enormously beneficial to the body, because they are jam-packed with nutrients and prevent spikes in blood sugar levels. Other forms of complex carbohydrates are starchy vegetables (also nutrient dense and loaded with fiber), like sweet potatoes, yams, and parsnips, as well as vegetables like broccoli, bell peppers, cauliflower, and spinach. The difference between all these types of complex carbohydrates that's valuable to know in relationship to body transformation and weight loss is that they vary on the Glycemic Index, a system that measures foods on a scale from 1–100 based on their effect on blood sugar levels. If weight loss is your goal, it is suggested you stick to eating complex carbohydrates that are low (less than 55) on the Glycemic Index, such as broccoli, bell peppers, lettuce, and mushrooms. Anything over 70 is considered high. We'll discuss the Glycemic Index in more detail later in this appendix.

Complex carbohydrates are also essential to the body because they aid in healthy body composition transformation, help to lower blood cholesterol, reduce the risk of heart disease, support the nervous system, and help aid in healthy bone growth. Omitting all carbohydrates from your diet is a bad idea and not recommended.

Complex carbohydrates take longer for the body to break down and digest than simple carbs (which we'll get to in a minute), so they deliver a gradual supply of glucose to the bloodstream. *Glucose* is the most essential source of energy for your body and is used to fuel your body for normal daily activity and exercise. When glucose is delivered slowly and steadily to the cells, it provides sustained energy, helps maintain normal blood sugar levels, and keeps your mood stable. It also provides a steady stream of energy during your workouts and why it's recommended to consume a large percentage of your daily carbohydrate consumptions prior to exercising.

Simple carbohydrates, on the other hand, are *not* good for the body and, generally speaking, should be minimally consumed or omitted from the diet as much as possible. Simple carbohydrates come in the form of sugars, whereas complex carbohydrates come in the form of starches and fiber. With the exception of fiber, which is not absorbed by the body, all carbohydrates are converted into glucose or sugar during digestion. Simple carbs are easy for your body to break down, so they are absorbed quickly and cause a fast spike in blood sugar levels. White sugar, white flour, candy, syrups, sugar-sweetened soft drinks, alcoholic beverages, and all fruits are all examples of simple carbohydrates. While fruits are a great source of antioxidants for the body, we do need to be aware of their sugar amounts.

When you eat a lot of simple carbohydrates, the excess sugar floods your system and because your body is not able to use it all for energy, it ultimately converts the sugar to fat which gets dumped into your liver and various other parts of the body for later use—which never comes. Consumption of high levels of sugar can cause diseases like diabetes and hypoglycemia and of course obesity.

On the other hand, because simple carbohydrates require little digestion, they can be a quick source of energy as part of a post-workout meal. When coupled with some protein, they can assist the body to more rapidly absorb the protein it needs to build and repair the muscles just trained. This is why athletes will often drink a protein shake that either includes a high GI food source or add to their protein high GI foods like banana. The only healthy simple carbohydrate you should be consuming is fruit in moderation, because fruit provides some valuable nutrients and antioxidants that fight off free radicals, protect the immune system, and prevent disease. But the key is definitely moderation if fat loss is your goal. When weight loss is your goal, I suggest reducing your carbs intake to 45 percent or less of your daily calories from carbs, and to pay close attention to how your body responds to your levels of activity. However this is based on my personal and professional experience. The following is the daily carbohydrate recommendation from the Mayo Clinic (http://www.mayoclinic.org/how-to-eat-healthy/ART-20046590): "Emphasize natural, nutrient-dense carbohydrates from fruits and vegetables, beans and legumes, and whole grains. Limit less healthy sugar-sweetened beverages, desserts, and refined grain products. Get 45 to 65 percent of your daily calories from carbohydrates. Carbohydrates have 4 calories a gram. Based on a 2,000-calorie-a-day diet, this amounts to 900 to 1,300 calories a day, or about 225 to 325 grams."

A Word about Fiber

Often referred to as "roughage," fiber is also an important element in your diet that's valuable for you to know about. Fiber supports the digestive process, helps to combat constipation, is thought to lower the bad cholesterol, possibly prevents against some forms of cancers, can protect against heart disease, and can aid in regulating blood-sugar levels. There are two basic types of fiber: insoluble and soluble. Insoluble fibers include foods such as whole grains and vegetables and can assist to prevent constipation. Soluble fibers include foods like oats and apples and assist with improving blood sugar levels and cholesterol.

Here is the Mayo Clinic daily fiber recommendation (http://www.mayoclinic.org/how-to-eat-healthy/ART-20046590): "Emphasize whole-grain products, fruits, vegetables, beans and peas, and unsalted nuts and seeds. If you're a woman, get about 22 to 28 grams of fiber a day. If you're a man, get about 28 to 34 grams of fiber a day."

The Skinny on Fats

Dietary fat is a controversial subject these days. There are different types of fats, and it is generally acknowledged by everyone that trans fats (also known as hydrogenated fats) are unhealthy, and unsaturated fats—both monounsaturated and polyunsaturated—have huge health benefits and are in fact necessary for the healthy functioning of the entire body. It is the subject of saturated fats that causes debate. It is commonly believed that saturated fats are bad and to be avoided, but more recent research has shown that there are significant health benefits to be gained from eating a certain amount of saturated fat, which can be found in foods like avocados, nuts, and organic salmon.

The right type of fats are beneficial to the body because dietary fat assists your body in absorbing essential vitamins that support the function and structure of cell membranes as well as your immune system. Fat also helps keep you satiated (feeling full), and while fat has more calories (9 calories a gram, versus carbohydrates and proteins, which both have 4 calories a gram), it is essential to include fat in your diet on a daily basis.

Here is the daily fat recommendation from the Mayo Clinic (http://www.mayoclinic.org/how-to-eat-healthy/ART-20046590): "Emphasize unsaturated fats from healthier sources, such as lean poultry, fish, and healthy oils, such as olive, canola, and nut oils. Limit [or better yet, omit completely] less healthy full-fat dairy products, desserts, pizza, burgers, sausage, and other fatty meats. To keep fat at bay, limit all sources of fat to 20 to 35 percent of your daily calories. Fat has 9 calories a gram. Based on a 2,000-calorie-a-day diet, this amounts to about 400 to 700 calories a day, or about 44 to 78 grams of total fat."

The Skinny on Protein

Protein is also essential to the body, because you need protein in your diet to build muscle and burn fat. These days many people aren't eating enough protein, which significantly contributes to weight problems and obesity. Eating protein will help you sustain a healthy immune system, repair and maintain tissue such as bones and skin, support the nervous system, and help your body make and repair cells. Dietary protein is an essential nutrient made of complex organic compounds called amino acids. Foods that contain all nine essential amino acids are called *complete proteins*. These foods include anything derived from animal sources, such as beef, chicken, fish, eggs, milk, yogurt, butter, and cheese. Soybeans are the only plant protein considered to be a complete protein.

Incomplete proteins have a deficiency of one or more of the nine essential amino acids. Sources of incomplete proteins include beans, lentils, peas, nuts, seeds, oats, wheat, pasta, and rice. Incomplete proteins, like rice and beans, can be combined to form a complete protein. This is how vegetarians and vegans can stay healthy and support the proper functioning of their bodies without eating meat or dairy. Generally speaking, two to three servings of a complete protein per day will meet the needs of most adults, but just as with the other macronutrients, I suggest my clients pay attention to their body's responses and make changes and modifications where necessary. Every body is different. I consume sometimes 5 or more protein servings a day; some people can consume and process protein more easily than others.

The Mayo Clinic's daily protein recommendation is as follows (http://www.mayoclinic.org/how-to-eat-healthy/ART-20046590): "Emphasize plant sources of protein, such as beans, lentils, soy products, and unsalted nuts. These high-protein foods have the added bonus of being higher in health-enhancing nutrients than are animal sources of protein. Eat seafood twice a week. Meat, poultry, and dairy products should be lean or low fat. Get 10 to 35 percent of your total daily calories from protein. Protein has 4 calories a gram. Based on a 2,000-calorie-a-day diet, this amounts to about 200 to 700 calories a day, or about 50 to 175 grams a day."

Understanding Micronutrients

Micronutrients are only needed by the body in small amounts and are made up of vitamins (vitamin A, vitamin B, vitamin C, vitamin D, vitamin E, vitamin K, and carotenoids), trace minerals (boron, calcium, chloride, chromium, cobalt, copper, fluoride, iodine, iron, magnesium, manganese, molybdenum, phosphorous, potassium, selenium, sodium, and zinc), and organic acids (acetic acid, citric acid, lactic acid, malic acid, choline, and taurine).

Although micronutrients are only needed in small amounts, they are essential to the optimal functioning of the body. It is ideal to get all your micronutrients from natural food sources, but it is not always easy to eat only the most pure, natural, nutritionally rich foods, so I recommend augmenting your diet with high-grade, multivitamin and mineral supplements. I recommend that you consult with a registered dietician, nutritionist, naturopath, or integrative or holistic doctor to get an accurate assessment of your nutritional needs. You will need different supplements depending on your overall health, gender, and age.

What Are Vitamins?

Vitamins are essential for normal cell function, growth, and development and assist in forming bone and tissue. They also regulate metabolism and help convert protein, fat, and carbohydrates into energy. The four fat-soluble vitamins, A, D, E, and K, are digested and absorbed with the help of fats in our diet and are stored in the body's fatty tissue. The water-soluble vitamins include the vitamin B group and vitamin C. They are not stored in the body for very long, and excess quantities are eliminated through the urine. Vitamin B12 is the only exception to that rule and can be stored in the liver for many years.

Vitamin A

Vitamin A is fat-soluble and helps maintain healthy bones, teeth, body tissues, skin, eyesight, and mucous membranes of the mouth, nose, throat, and lungs. It also supports the immune system and is involved in the synthesis of the hormone progesterone. The best sources for vitamin A are liver, eggs, dairy products, and dark green, yellow, and orange fruits and vegetables.

Vitamin B1 (Thiamine)

Vitamin B1 is water-soluble and is essential for growth, heart function, healthy muscles, and a healthy nervous system. It also helps with carbohydrate and amino acid metabolism. The best sources of vitamin B1 are yeast, legumes, wheat germ, nuts, whole grains, dried beans, eggs, seafood, and red meat.

Vitamin B2 (Riboflavin)

Vitamin B2 is water-soluble and is important for body growth. It is involved in the production of some enzymes, as well as the production of red blood cells. The best sources of vitamin B2 are yeast, wheat germ, whole grains, green leafy vegetables, broccoli, dairy, eggs, lean meats, and liver.

Vitamin B3 (Niacin)

Vitamin B3 is water-soluble and helps promote healthy skin and keeps the digestive and nervous systems in good working order. It also helps with carbohydrate, fat, and protein metabolism, appetite regulation, and blood circulation. Good sources of vitamin B3 include meats, fish, legumes, nuts, whole grains, yeast, coffee, and tea.

Vitamin B5 (Pantothenic acid)

Vitamin B5 is water-soluble and is essential for nerve function and the metabolism of food. It also plays a role in the production of hormones and cholesterol. The best sources of vitamin B5 are lean meats, liver, whole grains, legumes, yeast, and green vegetables.

Vitamin B6

Vitamin B6 is water-soluble and helps support a healthy nervous system, maintain brain function, and form red blood cells. It also helps with protein and carbohydrate metabolism. The best sources for vitamin B6 are fish, poultry, lean meat, liver, yeast, potatoes, tomatoes, whole grains, and vegetables.

Vitamin B7 (Biotin)

Vitamin B7 is water-soluble and is essential for cell growth and the production of cholesterol, hormones, and fatty acids. It also promotes the metabolism of proteins, fat, and carbohydrates, is helpful in maintaining a healthy blood sugar level, and has been shown to strengthen hair and nails. Biotin is found in foods such as liver, egg yolk, dairy products, soybeans, yeast, legumes, nuts, and dark green vegetables.

Vitamin B9 (Folate or Folic acid)

Vitamin B9 is water-soluble and helps with red blood cell formation and protein metabolism, and is essential for the production of DNA. The best sources of Folate are poultry, liver, nuts, beans, whole grains, green leafy vegetables, and fruits.

Vitamin B12

Vitamin B12 is water-soluble and helps maintain the central nervous system. It also helps with the production of red blood cells, along with carbohydrate, fat, and protein metabolism. Vitamin B12 is found only in animal protein, and the best sources are red meat, liver, fish, poultry, eggs, and dairy products.

Vitamin C (ascorbic acid)

Vitamin C is water-soluble and promotes wound healing, healthy teeth, gums, bones, ligaments, blood vessels, and body tissues. It is also boosts the immune system, improves absorption of iron, and is needed for the synthesis of collagen. The best sources of vitamin C are citrus fruits, tomatoes, berries, melons, and green vegetables.

Vitamin D

Vitamin D is fat-soluble and is the only vitamin that can be produced by the human body. It helps the body absorb calcium, which is needed for the development and maintenance of healthy bones and teeth. Vitamin D is made by the body after being in the sun. The best sources of vitamin D, aside from sunshine, are eggs, fatty fish, fish liver oil, and enriched milk. In countries with less sunshine (like Canada), vitamin D is essential to good health and low vitamin D levels have been linked to weight and other health issues.

Vitamin E (tocopherol)

Vitamin E is fat-soluble and promotes red blood cell formation, helps maintain healthy oxygen levels in membranes and DNA, and aids the body in using vitamin K. It also plays a role in immune function, protects tissues from damage, and as an antioxidant, reduces the risk of heart disease and cancer. The major sources of vitamin E are dark green vegetables, seed oils, palm and rice oils, wheat germ, whole grains, nuts, sunflower seeds, beans, eggs, and liver.

Vitamin K

Vitamin K is fat-soluble and makes the proteins that allow blood to clot, and vitamins K and D together support bone strength. Vitamin K also keeps calcium out of the arteries and helps keep the linings of blood vessels in a flexible condition. The best sources of vitamin K are green leafy vegetables, alfalfa, beef liver, vegetable oils, cauliflower, soybeans, kiwi, and avocadoes.

The Power of Leafy Greens

Organic leafy greens and vegetables are chock full of vitamins (A, C, K, E, and some B vitamins), minerals (including calcium, potassium, iron, and magnesium) and dietary fiber! According to the latest studies, the nutrients found in dark, leafy greens, and vegetables may prevent cancer, heart disease, and diabetes, as well as boost the immune system, increase bone strength, promote eye health, aid digestion, and facilitate weight loss.

In addition to being high in nutritional value, leafy vegetables are low in calories and low on the glycemic index, which means you can fill up on them without worrying about gaining weight! Leafy greens and vegetables can even be considered "negative calorie foods," as it takes as many calories for you to digest them as you get out of eating them. The high amounts of fiber in leafy greens will suppress your appetite and curb your sugar cravings while aiding in detoxification of the body by regulating the digestive system and promoting elimination. So fill up that salad bowl with a variety of fresh, organic greens and veggies, and dig in!

Lettuce is high in vitamins A, C, K, and folic acid. The darker the lettuce leaf, the more nutritional value it has.

Spinach is high in vitamins A, C, K, E, riboflavin, thiamin, niacin, and folic acid, as well as the mineral iron. You get more nutritional value out of cooked spinach because heating it frees up its dietary calcium.

Arugula has a peppery flavor and is high in vitamins A and C, and the mineral calcium.

Broccoli is high in vitamins C, A, and folic acid, as well as the mineral potassium.

Cabbage is an excellent source of vitamin C.

Kale is a terrific source of vitamins A, C, K, and folic acid, as well as calcium and potassium.

Swiss chard has a slightly bitter, beet-like flavor and is a great source of vitamins A, C, K, E, folic acid, niacin, biotin, and pantothenic acid. It is also an excellent source of zinc, calcium, magnesium, phosphorous, manganese, copper, potassium, and iron.

Collards greens are similar to kale in their nutritional makeup.

Turnip greens are somewhat sharp in flavor but high in vitamins A, C, and K, as well as calcium.

Mustard greens have a peppery taste and are similar to turnip and collard greens in their nutritional makeup.

Bok Choy is a Chinese white cabbage high in vitamins A and C and calcium.

Dandelion greens taste a little sharp and spicy but are full of vitamin A and calcium.

Staying Hydrated: Helpful Information about Water

How much water should you drink each day? The amount of water you need has to do with your environment, your health, your weight, your gender, whether you are pregnant or breast-feeding, and how active you are. The Institute of Medicine, which is the health arm of the National Academy of Sciences, recommends that a healthy adult woman, living in a temperate climate, should drink approximately 9 cups of water a day, and a healthy man should drink approximately 13 cups a day.

Some health experts believe that you can determine the amount of water you need daily by dividing your weight in pounds by half. That number represents the number of ounces you should drink in a day. For instance, if you weigh 180 pounds, you should drink about 90 ounces or 11 ¼ cups of water daily.

In order to avoid dehydration, you should drink water *before* you're thirsty. By the time you're feeling thirsty, you are already dehydrated. Even mild dehydration can cause headaches, muscle and joint pains, and constipation. Another sign to look for is in your urine. If your urine is dark yellow, you are not drinking enough water.

In general, my recommendation is to drink water consistently throughout the day and keep a bottle of water with you at all times. In particular, have a bottle of water to sip on when you're exercising. I drink 2–3 liters of water a day. If you get tired of the taste of plain water, add a squeeze of fresh lemon, lime, or orange, or prepare a pitcher of water with fresh, crushed mint and cut cucumbers, and put in the refrigerator to drink when cold. If you drink alcohol (which is dehydrating), drink one glass of water for each glass of alcohol to stay adequately hydrated. Where possible, drink from glass, not plastic. Plastic contains chemicals known to be detrimental to your health, causing hormonal imbalances as well as certain types of cancer. Again, employing the practice of mindfulness will help you discern how much water *your* body needs.

Calories

When you're standing in front of the Starbucks counter looking over the pastries and muffins, and you choose to buy a 400-calorie slice of lemon cake, that calorie amount represents how much energy your body will get from eating the cake. But what your body does with the calories is another story, as not all calories are created equal.

A calorie is, very simply, a unit of energy. I'm sure you've heard the term "empty calories" and have maybe wondered what that means. Your body will process the refined sugar, white flour, and fat in that lemon cake differently than it would process 400 calories of salad made with organic, leafy greens; an organic, chopped, hard-boiled egg; a sprinkling of sunflower seeds; chicken breast; and good virgin olive oil.

The cake's calories, which are primarily sugar and nutrient deficient, will spike your blood sugar, making you feel energetic temporarily, and then making you crash hard. When you crash, you will feel irritable, depleted, and hungry again. It's a vicious cycle. The salad, on the other hand, is nutrient dense and will give you a more constant, stable level of energy, so you'll feel better and be more productive over the long haul. The "empty calories" in the cake will be converted to stored fat, while the calories in the salad will give you the "get up and go" to optimize the energy from those calories, which will ultimately help you lose weight.

So the body needs energy in the form of calories to function, but all calories are not created equal. This is precisely why I never advocate calorie counting as the definitive answer to weight loss. It is fine to be aware of calorie intake versus energy expenditure (activity), but more important is to be aware of the quality of the food you eat (whether it is nutrient dense or not) and the physiological feelings and responses you get after eating it. Another issue with counting calories exclusively as a way to lose weight is that the amount of calories needed varies from person to person and day to day, depending on how much energy you are expending. Counting calories just isn't necessary when we are paying close attention to our body, nor is it a lot of fun. Who wants to count calories all day long? Therefore, in my opinion, calorie counting is not a natural process, and it can even be unhealthy if we aren't aware of the quality of our calories.

I like what wellness consultant and author of *The Fast Metabolism Diet,* Haylie Pomroy, has to say about calories: "The calories in/calories out theory is a vast and grossly deceiving oversimplification of how the body uses energy. It is also, in my opinion, a malicious marketing tool that has been used to advocate unhealthy and damaging foods."[28]

Pomroy also goes on to say, and I agree with her wholeheartedly, that "each person has a unique body and biochemical make-up—so a calorie isn't going to be the same thing for you as it is for anyone else."[29] Pomroy also states, and I paraphrase here, that every different body has a different way of metabolising and distributing the energy derived from food. Some bodies may *store* fat from eating a lettuce leaf, whereas another body may shed fat.[30] Suffice to say, calorie counting is not something I recommend adopting as a temporary habit or a lifestyle.

Although I'm not an advocate of calorie counting as a way to lose weight, I do adhere to the recommendation of the American College of Sports Medicine (ACSM) that calorie consumption should never drop below 1200 calories per day for women, or 1800 calories per day for men.

The Glycemic Index

The Glycemic Index (GI) ranks carbohydrates on a scale from 0–100, according to their effect on blood glucose (or blood sugar) levels in the body and provides another important piece of information to know about when learning about nutrition and changing your body composition. Pure glucose or sugar is ranked at 100. High GI foods are rated at greater than 70, moderate GI foods are rated between 56–69, and low GI foods are rated at less than 55. High GI foods are quickly digested and absorbed into the bloodstream and result in a spike in blood sugar levels. Lower GI foods are digested more slowly and release glucose into the bloodstream more gradually. As previously mentioned, low to moderate GI foods are best consumed the majority of the time if fat loss and maintenance of a healthy body composition is the goal.

What Is Blood Sugar?

Blood sugar refers to the amount of sugar (glucose) in the blood. Glucose, remember, is the main source of energy for the body and is delivered to the cells through the bloodstream. The hormone insulin, which is produced in the pancreas, makes glucose available for utilization by the body. A consistently high blood sugar level is called *hyperglycemia*, and a consistently low level is called *hypoglycemia*. People with diabetes have high blood sugar levels, or hyperglycemia, and if not treated, may experience stroke, heart disease, kidney disease, vision problems, and nerve damage. The symptoms of chronically low blood sugar, or hypoglycemia, may include lethargy, shaking, weakness, diminished mental ability, and in extreme instances, brain damage, coma, or death.

How Are Blood Sugar Levels Managed within the Body?

Glucose in the bloodstream rises about one hour after a meal. The pancreas detects high levels of glucose in the blood and secretes insulin. Insulin encourages the liver and muscles to absorb glucose out of the blood causing blood glucose levels to drop back to normal.[31]

Why Is a Low GI Diet Desirable?

Foods with a low GI are generally more nutritious and higher in fiber than high GI foods. Because they are absorbed by the body more gradually, they help you feel fuller for a longer period of time, which means you may be less likely to overeat. Higher GI foods are metabolized by the body quickly, which can make you hungry again sooner. They also cause a spike in blood sugar, which induces your pancreas to secrete more insulin, causing the excess sugar to be converted to stored fat. The extra insulin released to metabolize the high GI foods may initially make you feel more energized, but it will ultimately drive your blood sugar down too low, causing a drop in your energy level, or a sugar crash.

So you could keep reaching for your mid-afternoon cookie (high GI) and end up feeling fat and more tired than ever, or you can make a healthier choice by eating something like cucumber slices with a handful of almonds, which will give you a more stable energy level for a longer period of time. By paying attention to the glycemic values of the foods you eat, you can design a diet to achieve optimal blood sugar levels.

Overall, eat less processed and refined foods, and eat more whole grains, lean proteins, vegetables, and fruits. High-glycemic foods to avoid are all foods with high sugar content (candy, cookies, cake), all foods prepared with refined white or wheat flour (bread, crackers, pancakes, pasta), and all sugary soft drinks.

Again, there are some times when eating higher glycemic foods is beneficial, such as after strenuous exercise in combination with a protein source to aid in recovery. However, lower glycemic foods are generally recommended for maintaining stable blood sugar levels and promoting overall good health, and you should always select natural higher glycemic foods for post-workout meals, like a banana.

To learn more about the Glycemic Index and GI Database, which will help you determine the GI value of any food, visit www.glycemicindex.com.

CONTINUE YOUR TRANSFORMATION JOURNEY

To download a free audio meditation developed by Michelle …
www.michellearmstrong.com/transformbook

ABOUT THE AUTHOR

Michelle Armstrong is a "next-generation thought leader," bestselling author, fitness trainer, holistic health practitioner, motivational coach and speaker, and the creator of the Renovate Your Life programs and events.

Michelle has numerous credentials in the fields of psychology, metaphysics, spirituality, bioenergetics, nutrition, health, and fitness. She has privately coached and trained more than 700 individuals and spoken to thousands worldwide.

Michelle is passionate about empowering people to live their best life. She has a profound ability to rapidly connect with people at a very deep level and identify the areas within their minds that are holding them back from reaching their full potential. She teaches people how they can change their life circumstances and get the results they want by changing their mental blueprint through her practices of mindful and emotional awareness, faith, and her unique practices and methods.

Michelle coaches and works with small businesses and large corporations, professional athletes and performers, fitness professionals, entrepreneurs and leaders, and anyone striving to be their best in life. She is also passionate about giving back and linking arms with other inspiring and motivating leaders.

When Michelle isn't traveling the world sharing her messages or working privately with her clients, she loves to write, play with her son, listen to music, sing, meditate, pray, laugh with her friends, and lift weights. Originally from Down Under, Michelle now lives in Canada.

ENDNOTES

1   Bruce Lipton, *The Biology of Belief* (Hay House, 2005).

2   Ibid.

3   Ibid.

4   Ibid.

5   Neville Goddard, *The Power of Awareness* (DeVorss & Company, 1952, revised 1992).

6   Bruce Lipton, *The Biology of Belief* (Hay House, 2005), xv.

7   Gregg Braden, *The Spontaneous Healing of Belief* (Hay House, 2008), xiv, 53.

8   Michael Talbot, *The Holographic Universe* (HarperCollins, 1992), 6.

9   Bernie S. Siegel, *Love, Medicine, and Miracles* (HarperCollins, 1986).

10 Eckhart Tolle, *A New Earth: Awakening to Your Life's Purpose* (Penguin, 2005), 96.

11 Eckhart Tolle, *The Power of Now* (Namaste Publications, 1999), 24.

12 Louise Hay, *Heal Your Body* (Hay House, 1982), 3.

13 To learn more about our food cravings and what they can tell us about our moods, see Doreen Virtue, *Constant Craving: What Your Food Cravings Mean and How to Overcome Them* (Hay House, 2005).

14 Hay, *Heal Your Body*, 54.

15 James Colquhoun and Laurentine Ten Bosch, *Food Matters* (video), Permacology Productions, 2008, www.foodmatters.tv/.

16 Colquhoun and Ten Bosch, *Food Matters*.

17 According to the Health Canada's Dietary Reference Intakes Tables, "No required role for these nutrients [saturated fats] other than as energy

sources was identified; the body can synthesize its needs for saturated fatty acids and cholesterol from other sources." See http://www.hc-sc.gc.ca/fn-an/nutrition/reference/table/index-eng.php.

18 The World Health Organization has a similar recommendation: no more than 5 percent of daily calories should come from sugar, or the equivalent of 6 teaspoons. "Lower sugar intake to less than 5% of daily calories, WHO says," CBC News, March 5, 2014, http://www.cbc.ca/news/health/lower-sugar-intake-to-less-than-5-of-daily-calories-who-says-1.2560639.

19 Colquhoun and Ten Bosch, *Food Matters.*

20 Colquhoun and Ten Bosch, *Food Matters.*

21 Mary V. Gold, "Organic Production/Organic Food: Information Access Tools," Alternative Farming Systems Information Center, National Agricultural Library, United States Department of Agriculture, http://www.nal.usda.gov/afsic/pubs/ofp/ofp.shtml, accessed February 5, 2014.

22 Melissa Valliant, "Do Juice Cleanses Work? 10 Truths about the Fad," *The Huffington Post,* March 22, 2012, http://www.huffingtonpost.ca/2012/03/22/do-juice-cleanses-work_n_1372305.html, accessed November 1, 2013.

23 Melissa Valliant, "Do Juice Cleanses Work?"

24 Deepak Chopra, *Overcoming Addiction* (Three Rivers Press, 1997), 86-87.

25 Joel Fuhrman, "Redefining Hunger Can Kickstart Weight Loss," The Blog, *The Huffington Post,* December 5, 2010, http://www.huffingtonpost.com/joel-fuhrman-md/redefining-hunger_b_789980.html, accessed November 1, 2013.

26 Fuhrman, "Redefining Hunger Can Kickstart Weight Loss."

27 Mayo Clinic, "Hyperthyroidism," http://www.mayoclinic.org/diseases-conditions/hyperthyroidism/basics/definition/con-20020986.

28 Haylie Pomroy, *The Fast Metabolism Diet* (Harmony, 2013), 23.

29 Ibid.

30 Ibid.

31 Source: *Canadian Fitness Professional Nutrition and Wellness Specialist Manual.*

CPSIA information can be obtained at www.ICGtesting.com
Printed in the USA
LVOW06s2312230815

451200LV00011B/777/P

9 781630 473723